SECRET ASSASSINS IN FOOD

The Ninjas of Taste

Americans are under covert 'chemical' attack daily.
These chemicals are affecting our brains and may well destroy our
society!

Shocking? Of course, but
What you don't know, can indeed kill you.
Big Business Buries the Truth and Silences the Majority.

Forewarned is Forearmed.

By A. True Ott, PhD
Contributions by Linda K. Hegstrand, MD, PhD
Forward by Wayne Pickering, N.D., Sc.M.

I

This Book is Dedicated to Chip, a fighter to the end,
All Truth Seekers and all who are Honest in Heart.
For You, every Day is a New Adventure.

And to Joan, the One Who Makes It All Happen

Special Thanks to Linda, Kelly, Mel, Gary, Randy, and Hundreds of Friends who have Caught the Vision of a World Free of Brain Warping, Inorganic Chemicals.

And to cartoonist Jeff Parker, whose gift is making us laugh, while he gently shows Americans the Truth.

Together, we can indeed CHANGE THE WORLD!

ISBN # 0-9764020-0-9

Cover designed by Jeremy T. Ott

Foreword

Since the 5 major killers in our country - Heart Disease; Cancer; Stroke; Diabetes & Obesity are all nutritionally related, if we corrected our eating habits then it would stand to reason we wouldn't have to worry so much about these problems. Age surely doesn't cause any of them; if that was the case then everyone who's old would be sick and we know for an absolute fact that this is just not true. www.HealthAtLast.com

Most of us give up on our health in our quest for wealth only to spend ALL that accumulated wealth just to try and regain our health. I've been counseling for years and I'm always encouraging people to make their health their first concern and not their last resort.

We are only here for a short time and with all the efforts we put into all other areas of our lives, it would be prudent to make health a top priority; for when we die, our brother-in-law gets to drive the car that we sacrificed our health and lives to buy in the first place.

When I was asked to write the forward to this incredible "must read" wealth of information, **"Secret Assassins in Food"** I was overjoyed as it always great to acknowledge those who are speaking and writing about the pure simple truth regarding this subject of **Food**.

Being sick and bedridden for months at a time several times in my life I knew that this was not for me. Life is a joy to be lived and not some problem to be solved all the time. So after I came back from the Viet Nam War (serving 3 tours of duty) I saw so much unhealthiness around me that I knew I had to do something about it.

I met an elderly lady who owned a health food store where I relocated for a short time after the war. She was real godsend to me, and changed my life. She gave me a book on how to be healthy by eating natural foods. It was so elementary, but it gave me the incentive to really look into the food I consumed in my life. Since then, I have literally made it a science. (See www.DefeatingBadEating.com)

I only wished I would have been exposed to such a wealth of information in this well documented book *"Secret Assassins in Food"* when I was suffering from all that horrible sickness such as Heart Problems; Labored Breathing; Horrific Indigestion; Plaguing Colds; a constant Weight Problem and the list goes on. Now I'm totally FREE of all of these debilitating conditions, NEVER knowing I was the one causing it all right from the beginning.

Since nobody likes change except a wet baby, I didn't want to make the changes until I absolutely had to. And lo and behold, it was so much easier when I wanted to than when I had to. If you will only eliminate the 3 foods to avoid at all cost (White Foods; Fizzy Foods; & Greasy Foods) in your diet and combine your foods properly, you will be amazed at the level of health you will take pleasure in. See www.HealthAtLast.com

Just from implementing the truths found in this book you may enjoy:

- LESS Body Fat; MORE Energy; Skin Problems DISAPPEARING…
- Medical Bills being DRASTICALLY REDUCED!
- IMPROVED Digestion; Your Clothes fit Better; Sweeter smelling Breath!
- A Sharpened Attitude; Improved Circulation & Better Muscle Tone!
- LESS Nervous Tension!
- Boost your Immunity & Feel GREAT once again increasing your VITALITY!
- Take pleasure in a good night's sleep and cope with stress with ease and a host of other benefits.

I learned a great lesson in life that beliefs will only be beliefs as long as we have people out there to believe them. But TRUTH will always be Truth whether we believe it or not. And this well researched volume of scientific evidence exposed in **"Secret Assassins in Food"** is the pure and simple truth about what we are putting into our remarkable bodies.

It's altruistic that we are not garbage dumps with hairy lids. We are marvels of design with an awesome regenerating power that completely renews our body every 7 years.

➤ Every 2-3 days we have a new lining in the mouth.

➤ Every 5 Days our Intestinal Lining is Renewed

➢ Every 11 Days our Respiratory Lining is Renewed

➢ Every 15 Days all our White Blood Corpuscles are Replaced

➢ Every 120 Days all our Red Blood Corpuscles are Replaced

➢ Every 6 Months we have a Whole New Blood Stream

➢ Every 11 Months we have a Whole New Cell Structure

➢ Every 2 Years we have a Whole New Bone Structure

➢ Every 7 Years we have a Brand New Body

So if this is true and we know this is one of the marvels of the body, then why do we die? If we are constantly renewing ourselves, then why do we die? At this rate, then we should live on forever!

Well here is my answer born of research. We know that all cells die off and new ones are replaced every second of our life. But they are always copies of the original cell. If you take a document and got a copying machine and copy it, then make a copy from that copy and so on for 10 different sequences; notice how the 10th generation (copy) looks dismal at best.

Well this is what happens to the cells in our body. They become less pronounced as time goes on. But we can slow down their deterioration and keep them shining as long as possible when you adhere to the facts and principles in **"Secret Assassins in Food".** Please understand that we are all on the Road to Death, but there is just no need to jump in the Passing Lane.

In Brooklyn there is a hospital where people spend the rest of their lives waiting for a donor transplant. They actually have to wait for someone to die so they can live. They're called the "POLE PEOPLE" where they walk around all day long carrying a pole of medicine bags with several needles from those bags going into their bodies. To walk around the floor 7 times is their goal and you should see the horrible state of health they're in. It would make your hair cringe.

NEVER FORGET:
➢ A normal bladder has 10,000 gallons of fluid going through it in a lifetime.

➤ Your ears have 24,500 fibers in each ear just to hear the sound

➤ Your lungs have 600 million air pockets just to take the air into the blood stream.

➤ The outer Layers of the skin are renewed every 2-4 weeks

➤ We have over 60,000 miles of Blood Vessels in the body to keep us working… that's about 2 ½ times around the Globe and pumping enough blood in your entire lifetime to fill a freight train 25 miles long.

➤ Your fingernails grow at about the same rate that the Atlantic Ocean is widening.

➤ Did you know that if all the electronic energy in the hydrogen atoms of your body could be used that you could supply all the electrical needs of a large industrialized country for almost an entire week?

➤ The atoms of your body contain a potential energy of more than 11 million kilowatts per pound…that means that an average person by this estimate is worth more than $85 million dollars. Phooey on that person who told us that we were only worth $1.06 some years back.

➤ And all the atoms of your body sing ... that if you could tune into them, you would hear a perfect harmony.

In summation, there's more to you than meets the eye and there's no one else like you on the earth or has ever been like you. YOU ARE TRULY UNIQUE!

If all the cell information and the configuration of the components of your body were illustrated in one document, do you know that it would take **5 million pages** just to print out the complex genetic code of **just one single cell.**

Did you ever consider how perfectly your body is timed and controlled? How it maintains a normal temperature of 98.6 degrees? How the blood pressure is properly regulated and why you breathe an average of 16 times a minute and your heart beats 72 times a minute? How common food is digested chemically and the nutritive part is transformed into body tissue – bone and muscle; blood and skin; hair and nails – and properly distributed while wastes and poisons are eliminated with no ill effect?

You are special with a non-negotiable self-worth … you're a champ, not a chump... When you eat good stuff you WILL be tough!

Don't let Age be your Cage. You are a Marvel of Design who is healthy automatically by design and sick only by default. In this informative manuscript you will learn how to avoid all those diseases that plague us to such extent that more die each year of these 5 nutritionally related diseases then all the wars and famine combined.

Remember, it's all an ATTITUDE ... YOU CAN BE HEALTHY! And here is a poem I wrote several years ago about the subject of Attitude when it comes to taking care of your body.

If you have enough Fortitude
To develop an Attitude
Of sincere Gratitude
For your body's Magnitude
You will have an Aptitude
To reach a higher Latitude
For an ultimate Altitude

I'm Wayne Pickering N.D. (Naturopathic Doctor), Sc.M. (Masters of Science in Nutrition) and known to so many folks as "The Mango Man" = THE AMBASSADOR FOR HEALTH.

I have Authored 10 Health Guides; several C/D ROM's; 8 Books; 22 Audio Learning Programs; award winning Video Series titled "Is Your Diet A Riot", 32 Special Reports, 10 Herbal Teas; 10 Therapeutic Tinctures; over 200 Articles on Fitness & Nutrition, a weekly e-zine that goes out to over 12,000 opted in subscribers & 10 Health Systems all distributed in 37 countries!

I'm a Nutritional Performance Coach, Life Management Consultant & Disease Prevention Specialist ... An International Professional Speaker (Past President of the Nat'l Speakers Assn. in Florida) where I have spoken in five countries showing thousands of people how to enjoy life totally free of health problems caused by poor nutrition.

My prognosis was death at age 30. Now, at 57 years young, I have competed in 50 Triathlons and Biathlons winning many trophies as well as being a double nominee for the Healthy American Fitness Leader Award.

As a licensed Florida Nutrition Counselor whose programs are approved for continuing education credits by the Florida and Alabama State Boards of Pharmacy and most recently by the Florida Board of Dentistry and the founder of the Daytona Beach based **Center for Nutrition & Life Management, Inc.,** I can tell you this book, "**Secret Assassins in Food**" is a must read.

The primary reason Dr. Ott has written this book is to help parents guide their children into becoming healthy and happy adults. These are my goals as well - to help educate the general public. Dr. Ott shows the layman how specific toxins common in our food supply affects the developing brain.

There is little doubt that our children and grandchildren are at risk. In my vast experience as a nutritional health coach, I can say without reservation that we are what we eat. As Dr. Ott outlines in the pages of this book, when our children consume certain toxin substances in our foods, IQ's are reduced and test scores plummet.

The common sense facts presented by Dr. Ott could well be the answer to this very serious problem. Perhaps all the educational approaches to such societal problems are, very simply, "off-base".

I know that when we reflect on any society, tribal community, culture, race, etc. we always witness those who have the most influence over the people. Is it the Chiefs or the Medicine Men? We all know it is the Medicine Men. Why is this? It is because we all FEAR what we don't know. Therefore we will pay anyone to do the work for us or to patch us up at any cost. And most of that time the cost is really the shortening of the quality of our lives and the quantity of our years. We are finally designed to last 120 years totally free of disease.

And one more rather cynical approach to that is it's so much more profitable keeping the people sick than it is to change the entire system to being well. Dr. Ott's book is a clear twinging of the public conscience, and cannot be summarily dismissed by those who are wrongfully seeking financial gains from the increased use of these brain toxins, and who show little or no concern for the long-term damage their products are causing in American consumers.

My final comment is simply: Nutrition DOES NOT HEAL! Vitamins do not heal, medicine does not heal; herbs do not heal. The body is the only entity that heals when you give it a chance. The body is the hero. A very important factor in becoming truly well is that we only get well by what comes out of us and not by what goes into us.

Nutrition is nothing more than a series of 4 processes (Digestion, Absorption, Assimilation and Elimination) that the body employs to make Food materials for the body to use ... Nothing More And Nothing Less. So I encourage you to "EAT GOOD STUFF AND YOU WILL ALWAYS BE TOUGH!

Wayne Pickering, N.D., Sc.M. www.WaynePickering.com

Introduction

The Plot - Exposed and Identified

"We have met the enemy, and he is us!" --- Pogo

My name is A. True Ott. I have a Nutrition PhD. I make no claims on being the smartest man in America, but I do not consider myself by any means to be a "village idiot" either. I am a published author and lecturer, with two editions of my book, Wellness Secrets for Life – An Owner's Manual for the Human Body widely distributed across North America and the U.K. I tell you this, not to brag, but only to show how insidious and well-hidden "The Plot" truly is. I, as a nutritionist, should have known better – but I didn't. I was absolutely and completely fooled, and became a victim too, like millions of other naïve Americans. I don't know about you, but I personally don't like to be conned. Especially when the stakes in this game involve my most valuable and prized possession – my mental, physical, and spiritual health and well-being.

You see, I learned very early in my life that without good health and vitality, achieving wealth, fame and fortune becomes pretty well meaningless. As the couplet I wrote declares:

"We squander Health in search of Wealth;
We Work, We Toil, We Slave.
Then we squander Wealth in Search of Health,
and all We get is the Grave."

It seems foolish to me personally to maintain and protect our home, cars and other personal items with annual insurance premiums – while taking our health and vitality largely for granted – consuming any and all processed food items we find on the grocery store shelves. I, like hundreds of millions of other unsuspecting and trusting American consumers, wrongfully assumed that the U.S. Government's Food and Drug Administration would protect my family and myself from all harmful drugs and potentially poisonous additives in our daily food supply. In other words, as long as it was labeled correctly and under protective packaging – I believed my food was safe to consume. I have found out that this line of thinking is absolutely dangerous. I now clearly understand that the primary responsibility for my personal health and the quality and safety of the food I consume is mine, and mine alone. I can no longer have faith that my governmental "servants" will protect me. Either through ignorance or greed, or some insane combination of both – the fact remains that Americans have been victimized. It is time to blow the whistle. It is time to wake up and reverse the disease trends that threaten the very fabric of our society.

The story I tell in these pages is not fiction. It is fact, and is supported by literally hundreds of independent research documents that for some reason have heretofore been largely ignored by America's mainstream media. I will do my very best to tell this story in easy to understand language; and try to limit using highly technical terminology. My goal and desire is to give every man, woman and child in North America the opportunity to be able to comprehend the very real danger this nation is facing. I want them to understand "The Plot".

I want them to understand the fact that corporate America is driven primarily by the bottom-line profit figures. Lobbyists are paid to increase, or at the very least maintain corporate profits. In essence, that means Lobbyists in large part determine the decisions made by our governments. They have incredible influence in both major political parties in America. The reality is that lobbyists are the primary driving force in America today. Governmental policy is seldom decided without consulting un-elected leaders in Big Business. In fact, the truth is that all modern wars are fought primarily to further specific Big Money interests. The single largest Big Money interest in the world today is Oil. The second largest, and very closely related is Pharmaceuticals, and the medical cartel that they control. In fact, the same elite families account for and own these two Big Money interests that generate trillions of dollars of profits annually worldwide.

I understand that the truth is often very difficult for most people to accept. I have no doubt that many who read these pages will quickly dismiss the message as they rush to buy their Big Macs and Whoppers. These will be the same people who today are "secure" with their government 9 to 5 jobs, medical "benefit" plans, and retirement portfolios, and who hate to "rock the boat". These will be the very people whose obese children will someday be asked to pay America's health care debt and find meaningful answers to the rampant chronic illness plaguing the nation. Will it then be too late?

The cartel families mentioned earlier are very shrewd and very cunning. They know that if the American people ever learned the truth, the whole truth, and nothing but the truth; there would be a revolution. So they have successfully accomplished two of their prime objectives over the last 5 decades. They have very successfully generated a massive propaganda machine designed to do one very important thing: control public opinion. Secondly, the evidence shows that   the American public has indeed been covertly medicated with drugs hidden as "harmless" food additives. These hidden drugs, or "secret assassins" have been clinically proven to greatly reduce human being's cognitive reasoning skills, while causing unnatural weight gains! (Cognitive Reasoning is the ability to learn knowledge and apply it in clear, rational, logical thought processes. Historically, this is referred to as wisdom.) In short, Big Business Has Buried The Truth! Sadly, one thing Hitler and his Nazi Party proved to the world is that if you tell enough people a big lie forcefully enough, and often enough, linking it to religious dogma and national pride and fantasy, it soon becomes accepted as Truth. However, it is a lie nevertheless. In reality, the tragedy is that the big lie, masquerading as truth, is destroying people's ability to utilize their highest potentials, and society as a whole is the ultimate loser.

There is nothing inherently wrong, or "evil" with making a fair and honest profit of course. This is how people are rewarded for their labors. However, the truth is that most, if not all, FDA committees have a majority of members with large vested interests in the pharmaceutical and food industries. Moreover, approximately 60% of all medical "education" is funded by the pharmaceutical industry alone. Yes, what I am declaring is that the FDA and Medical Schools are clearly biased, and are motivated primarily by profit at the expense of truth and natural remedies. It is very much like asking the sly, hungry fox to guard the henhouse! The biggest obstacle in solving the problem is the inflated egos of the majority of this country's medical professionals. They believe they alone are taught "The Truth" by virtue of their diplomas backed by incontrovertible "scientific" research. The vast majority simply do not take the time to look outside the box, the box that their minds have been placed in. They are not willing to accept that often their "scientific research" is funded, conducted, and completely controlled by the same cartel that "educated" them in the first place. If honest medical professionals would only objectively examine the literature referenced in this book, I have no doubt they will come to the same conclusions I have. The Truth is simply the Truth. It is empirical and never changing. Facts are Facts. Propaganda can only confuse and disparage the issues of Truth, while it protects the profits of Big Business. This is why Big Business Buries The Truth! Often times they have to, in order to generate large profits!

The good news is that more and more licensed health care practitioners with pure and honest hearts are now stepping outside of the box. They are in fact realizing that there is something terribly wrong with the system. This is not so much because of any new book they have read, but rather they have come to realize that they can no longer afford to pay their malpractice insurance premiums. It i said that necessity is the mother of invention. I submit in this case, necessity is the father of changing paradigms.

Is the primary reason for skyrocketing malpractice premiums the "corrupt" American legal profession, as many MD's claim? Or is it actually due to the fact that millions of Americans have been crippled and/or killed because of the medical profession's mode of operation – which is to diagnose a disorder, then prescribe a chemical compound or two to mask the symptoms? All too often, more prescriptions are given to counteract the side effects the initial prescription caused, then over time more and more are added resulting in a downward spiral in health and eventual malpractice litigation. In this book I will present a powerful argument that "corrupt lawyers" have very little to do with skyrocketing malpractice rates. Rather, the problem is in fact the result of a health care system that is in dire need of massive reforms. The system needs to place a much greater focus on natural/holistic medicine combined with sound nutritional practices. This is my professional diagnosis and prescription, but Big Business Buries the Truth!

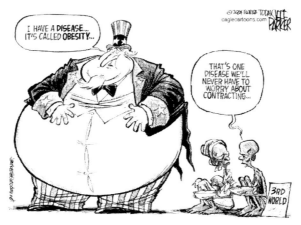

American "baby-boomers" are entering their middle age and approaching "senior" years – and the truth is, the vast majority (nearly 90%) of us are overweight.[i] According to statistics compiled by the National Institute of Diabetes & Digestive & Kidney Diseases, as of December 2001 – 58 Million Americans are classified as being overweight (10-30% over target weight for height), 40 Million are classified as "obese" (30-75% over target ideal weight), and 3 Million more are classified as "morbidly obese" (75% or more over ideal target weight).[ii] Let me clarify and restate – over 100 Million American adults are overweight. We are literally turning into a nation of sedentary couch potatoes – with incredible health challenges to face unless meaningful changes are made, and made quickly.

Did you also know that since 1990, there has been a 76% increase in Type II diabetes in 30-40 year old adults, and a full eight out of ten (80%) of Americans over the ripe old age of 25 are today classified as overweight.[iii]

If I still have not got your full attention, then consider this. A full 80% of Type II Diabetes is related to obesity, while 70% of Cardiovascular Disease (heart disease) is likewise directly related. 42% more breast cancers are diagnosed in obese women, while 26% of all overweight people have high blood pressure.[iv]

Worse yet, Obesity Related Disease (ORD) medical costs are beginning to overwhelm America's Health Care System – and are driving medical insurance rates through the roof. In short, even though you may be one of the small minority of people without a "weight problem" –('wait', you still have a problem) – you are having to pay the increased premiums just like your heavyweight friend.

When you consider that a full $63.14 **billion** was spent treating Type II Diabetes last year alone, while over $30 **billion** more was spent treating other obesity related disorders such as Heart Disease and Osteoporosis – this gives you some idea of the scope of the problem.[v] In addition to the cost of treatments, many billions of dollars worth of lost productivity also needs to be factored in.

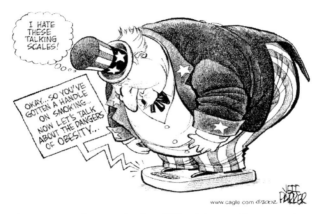

When I was growing up in the 60's, I honestly cannot remember too many overweight kids in my elementary school. Maybe 2 or 3, but rest assured, I could count them on the fingers of one hand. The national statistics report that in 1982, 4% of America's children were overweight. That number quadrupled to 16% just twelve years later in 1994. Seven years later, 1 out every 4 children (25%) in America aged 6-12 are overweight, and a full 33% of all African American and Hispanic children are overweight as of the year 2001.[vi] A new study suggests that 25% of these overweight children are already exhibiting early warning signs of type II Diabetes (impaired glucose tolerance testing), while over 60% already have at least one primary risk factor for heart disease.[vii] All of this before reaching puberty! Do you think this is a serious problem for America? What is going on? Are the children overweight because they are sedentary Nintendo/Game Cube junkies, or is there another reason, another link to "The Plot"??

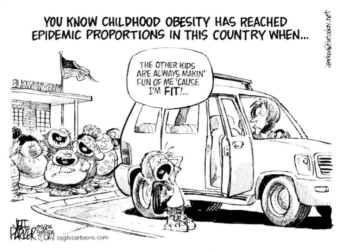

Consider that there are at least two other "disorders" growing in America's children at the same percentage rates as obesity; if you put your detective cap on, you may find a few clues that could help you find a suspect or two that may help to expose "the Plot". Specifically, the other two disorders are ADHD (Attention Deficit/Hyperactive Disorder) and Autism.   Both disorders exhibit rapidly growing statistics that strangely enough, mirror the increased percentages in juvenile obesity and diabetes.

If you are fortunate enough to have an elementary school educator for a personal friend, I am confident that she/he will tell you that Attention Deficit Hyperactive Disorder (ADHD) is preoccupying a lot of educators' and school boards' attention these days. One veteran educator confided to me that she believes that ADHD is rapidly becoming the most serious and prevalent problem with young students today. Hands down. No question about it. She may well be absolutely correct.

According to the National Institute of Mental Health (NIMH), a full 3% of American school children now have ADHD, and the number is growing rapidly.[viii] Like childhood obesity, ADHD has increased 500% in the last decade – and shows no signs of slowing down. If the causative factors to this trend are not identified and solutions applied, then by the year 2020, a full 75% of our school age children will be classified as Attention Deficit, and will be taking drugs such as Ritalin, Prozac, or Zoloft to "keep them on task." Many will be taking these brain drugs for life. The pharmaceutical giants must be licking their chops as they wait for the newest crop of sheep to arrive. Is it not time to pull the wool away from our eyes, and identify where the "big bad wolves" are hiding, if they do in fact exist? Or do we sit idly by and continue to allow our health to be compromised day by day? Is there a "silencing of the lambs" by means of subtle chemically induced frontal lobotomies? Do we keep "The Plot" unexposed, once it is discovered? Do we continue to allow Big Business to Bury the Truth? The decisions are yours to make. This book is written with the intent of helping you awaken to the truth of these very important issues.

Closely related biologically to ADHD is Autism, another form of mental disorder that is likewise growing in severity and occurrence. It is an ailment that manifests itself as the retardation of the mental abilities of the victim. Children diagnosed with the disorder exhibit extreme anti-social behavioral symptoms and are often abusive physically to themselves and others. Autistic children often exhibit abnormally low language development skills and may engage in repetitive physical motions. A few children diagnosed as Autistic have somewhat mild cases and can lead fairly normal lives. Others have exhibited advanced use of other areas of the brain, to the point where they are nothing short of genius. These are known as savants, as portrayed by Dustin Hoffman in the movie Rain Man. Savants are the ultimate paradox – they can have an extreme disability in one area such as speech or physical coordination, while at the same time exhibiting incredible ability and talents in other areas such as solving complex mathematical equations quickly and accurately, or mastering a musical instrument.

Autism statistics closely mirror those of ADHD. It was first named and discovered in the 1940's, and then only in isolated, extremely rare cases. Researchers found that it was genetic in nature, and developed in the unborn fetus during pregnancy. In other words, it was classified as a birth defect. Like ADHD, 75% of the individuals are male, 25% female. The key similarity however, is that the frequency of autism in births has increased 500% during the last decade, exactly like ADHD.

So, are the percentage increase similarities in obesity, ADHD, and autism just coincidental, or is there a central causative factor in all three? Does the Plot thicken – or does the law of statistics not apply? In other words, does lightning really strike the same foot of ground 3 times during the same thunderstorm?

At first, I didn't think the three were related. However, after reading Dr. Blaylock's Book, Excitotoxins – The Taste that Kills, and Dr. George Schwartz's Book, In Bad Taste, I began to do a little extended research into the subject. I uncovered a number of studies that clearly outlined the links between childhood obesity, ADHD, and Autism. Then I learned that this excito-toxic substance that is supposedly designed to make our food taste better, has also been placed in vaccines for infuenza, chickenpox, and MMR (measles, mumps, and rubella). I personally know of a number of parents who told me their children developed autism within days or weeks of receiving their vaccinations – and then I really began to wonder. Is this common food additive safe, or can it be highly dangerous, especially when directly injected into the bloodstream? Could this be an important, significant factor in adverse reactions to vaccinations, or are the reactions due mostly to other toxins found in vaccines, such as mercury? Moreover, could there possibly be a major problem with America's food supply because of the large amounts of this additive that are being consumed?

My research included any and all available international studies concerning Excito-toxins. I was stunned with the results of my research. Over 1000 different studies have been conducted worldwide on these man-made toxins. There are numerous maladies documented in humans and animals that consumed the substances. Symptoms often appear after only tiny dosages in some people. Could this common food additive be one of the primary causes in chronic diseases so widespread in North America today?

I found that pharmaceutical laboratories absolutely love this chemical, because it produces consistent, 100% reproducible results every time they use it. Specifically, this additive that is found in most processed food items in America, when injected under the skin of newborn mice and rats causes the rodents to grow obese well beyond their normal natural ranges.[ix] When it is injected directly into an experimental animal's brain, it quickly and efficiently kills the animal!! If this commonly used, chemical food additive does not fit the definition of a **poison**, then I do not know what does! Every person and every parent in America should be incensed and outraged by what is happening. I know I am.

I found that Drs. Olney, Schwartz, and Blaylock were absolutely correct. In my assessment, however, the dangers outlined in their books are grossly understated. Not only is this common food additive apparently a causative factor in gross obesity, autism and ADHD in our children, but is also linked to asthma, schizophrenia, gastro-intestinal disorders, lethargy, chest pains, migraine headaches, clinical depression, nausea, dizziness, uncontrollable rage reactions, and paranoia in the adult populations. Yet according the FDA, this chemical food additive can be added to any food in uncontrolled amounts.

Now I know that all Americans do indeed have a real problem. It appears that we are systematically being poisoned without our knowledge or consent. I cannot in good conscience sit idly by and do absolutely nothing about it. Once a person is warned, a good neighbor warns others. I wrote this book, and am beginning a new lecture circuit as my way of being a good neighbor. It is truly the most vital message of the 21st Century. For me, this knowledge and disseminating this information is now my life's mission.

---

[i] National Institute of Diabetes & Digestive & Kidney Diseases Report, Jan. 1, 2003

[ii] Ibid, Jan. 1, 2003

[iii] Ibid, Jan 1, 2003

[iv] Ibid, Jan. 1, 2003

[v] Ibid, Jan. 1, 2003

[vi] Tremblay MS, Williams JD, "Secular trends in the body mass index of children," CMAJ 2000; 163:1429-33

[vii] Ibid, Jan. 1, 2001

[viii] NIMH Report, ADHD and ADD Incidence in North America, Statistical Evaluation, Mar. 2002

[ix] Moss D. Ma., A. Cameron, DP. "Defective thermoregulatory thermogenesis in Monosodium Glutamate-induced obesity in mice." Metabolism 1985 Jul;34(7):626-30

Chapter 1

The Main Suspects

*All truths are easy to understand once they are discovered; the point
is to discover them.*
- Galileo Galilei

*The truth is incontrovertible. Malice may attack it, ignorance may
deride it, but in the end, there it is.*
- Winston Churchill

Throughout the various organs of the human body, as well as the
Central Nervous System (CNS) specifically the brain stem and frontal
lobes, you can find a number of specialized cells that are equipped
with various types of antennae-like appendages called glutamate
(amino acid) receptors.   These "glutamate receptors" work much like
specialized chemical sensors in a holding tank – when certain amino
acids like free glutamate become too abundant in and around the
organ's tissues, the receptor cells initiate a chain reaction in the
endocrine system and the brain to immediately produce specific
chemicals and hormones to safely absorb, or eliminate their toxic
effects as necessary. Some examples of these chemicals and
hormones are melatonin, serotonin, insulin, testosterone and
estrogen. In this process, protein molecules and minerals such as
calcium, magnesium, sodium, potassium, chromium, vanadium and
zinc are also utilized and literally hundreds of complex chemical
transmutations occur. The miracle is, this is all performed naturally
and quietly by the subconscious mind without the conscious brain

realizing what is happening. This is accomplished every second of every day. The incredible machine we call the human body is truly a priceless work of creation. But sadly, modern biochemical business products are short-circuiting the creator's brilliant natural design. Certain man-made chemical food additives have been added to processed food in toxic amounts, which causes the brain and endocrine system to produce an imbalance in specific brain chemicals. From a naturopathic worldview, any imbalance in the body translates into a disease condition, that modern medicine "treats" with yet another synthetic chemical drug. Millions of Americans are today suffering needlessly from these disease states. Meanwhile, pharmaceutical giants continue to reap the profits produced largely by the naivety and ignorance of the American public.

Neuroscientists have discovered that an amino acid called L-Glutamate produces a specific reaction in the human brain. It acts primarily as an excitatory substance, which means that it causes the brain to be electrically stimulated in much the same way that cocaine does. Using biochemical-mapping techniques, neuroscientists have proven that many key areas of the brain (such as the cortex, striatum, hippocampus, hypothalamus, thalamus, cerebellum and visual and auditory ear system) all contain an elaborate and extensive network of glutamate specific neurons.[i] In short, consumption of even small amounts of synthetic glutamates and aspartates can produce a wide variety of neurological and physical symptoms in certain individuals.

This book will show you how specific man-made, chemically produced acidic amino acids and peptides (specifically glutamates and aspartates) over-stimulate these special receptors, and as a result a number of brain functions concerned with sensory perception (vision and hearing), memory, orientation in time and space, cognitive reasoning, and motor skills are being negatively affected in literally millions of Americans. It is critical for the reader to understand that the human brain is an organ that is totally dependent upon a very delicate balance of excitatory and inhibitory signals, in other words, both positive and negative electrical impulses must be kept in a natural balance as long as possible. Even minor disruptions of this balance can lead to anything from a minor trembling of the hands, numbness in the extremities, or worse, to a full blown seizure in extreme cases. More often than not, however, these imbalances lead to subtle chemical and/or hormonal dysfunctions within the brain and various organs, and one of the first things disrupted are sleep cycles. To reach one's highest and best potential and live one's life to the fullest, understanding the importance of, and implementing wise dietary choices to achieve and maintain a balance between these positive and negative impulses is all important. In fact, its importance can simply not be overstated.

To stimulate the brain into un-natural cravings and food addictions, modern biochemists have genetically altered bacteria to produce specific amino acids. These unnatural, un-bound "free" amino acids fool the brain, and disrupt the brain's chemical balance. They are absorbed 8-10 times faster and in much larger numbers into the human bloodstream, often overpowering the glutamate receptors.

When these substances encounter the glutamate receptors on the specialized cells, the endocrine system in turn responds incorrectly – much like when a false address and false report is given to the dispatcher on a 911 emergency call. Valuable assets are misdirected, and taken away from areas where they are truly needed, or worse, they are so exhausted from the many false alarms that they have responded to, that they are not able to perform the job they specialize in when the real need arises. In time, the system begins to break down and fail. Chaos inevitably ensues. When this happens in the human body, chronic disease states are the unfortunate result. Disease states that have been linked to the consumption of large amounts of such manmade amino acids include diabetes, Creitzfeld-Jakob Disorder (CJD, human form of mad cow disease), Parkinson's disease, ADHD, autism, ALS (Lou Gehrigs's Disease), Alzheimer's, clinical depression, Bell's palsy, fibromyalgia, chronic fatigue syndrome, and of course, obesity and all obesity related diseases (ORDs).

In the last decade, it became painfully aware to most Americans that large tobacco companies place chemical stimulants onto the dried tobacco leaf prior to producing their cigarettes. The tobacco companies' marketing campaigns specifically targeted young teens with mind-manipulating ads during the 50's and 60's – equating smoking cigarettes with being macho, "popular" and "groovy". Once a teen began smoking, the addicting effects of the nicotine and added chemicals on the endocrine system took effect – and the teen was typically hooked for life – often a much shorter life, but that didn't really matter – the company's bottom line profit margin was increased by the teen's carton a week addiction. The added chemicals cause an unnatural brain chemistry reaction. The sad truth is that it took American society over 60 years to wake up and finally take the Industry to task – but that hasn't slowed it down much. They are now targeting other markets in developing 3rd world countries with a new crop of naïve consumers, and profits are steady. They are just not increasing at the preferred 15% per year growth rates that the manufacturers of chemically altered amino acid food additives have experienced over the last 3 decades!

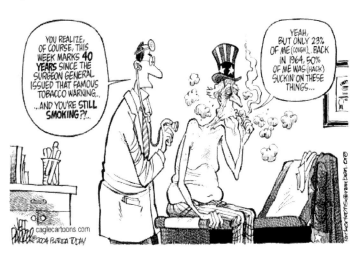

Cigarettes, however, have become a convenient target. Non-smokers have forcefully demanded their rights to clean air in restaurants and other public facilities. The polarity is clear-cut, and the health impacts now are plainly visible. But what if the health impacts of a specialized, addicting drug similar to nicotine are largely invisible, very subtly hidden, and yet is directly affecting the ENTIRE population of America while it is covertly and quietly added to the food we all consume and in the popular beverages we drink? Moreover, it appears this covert drugging is being done without the knowledge or consent of "we the people"! Should we blindly continue to ignore the warning signs until the nation is totally crippled mentally, financially and physically? Our other alternative is to make informed decisions based on facts, rather than on the profit-centered bottom-line and then require the nation's bureaucrats to do their job of protecting the public welfare with basic principles of integrity and honesty. This is not currently happening, and is yet another example where Big Business Buries the Truth.

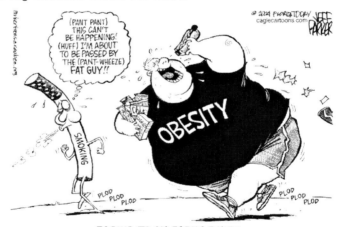

RACING TO AN EARLY FINISH...

To put the problem into perspective, what would be your reaction if you found out that a colleague at work was covertly spiking your food and drink daily with a chemical drug that made you gain weight rapidly while reducing your mental capacity and reaction times? What would be your response if you uncovered that he/she did this primarily with the intent to leap-frog over you and get the bigger office and higher salary because you were not as able to keep up and be competitive? In other words, he/she did it solely for personal financial and political gain! If this were in fact occurring, would you not greatly appreciate another colleague alerting you to the situation when he/she uncovered the truth?

In a very real sense, this is exactly what appears to be happening in America today. It appears we are being systematically drugged without our knowledge or consent, and this drug may be greatly diminishing our mental cognizance! There is little room for doubt that consuming this "Secret Assassin" chemical is directly related to the nation's obesity levels. Here's a real "news flash" America! We don't need to adopt an Atkin's or South Beach high protein diet in order to lose weight – we instead need to learn to read labels and eliminate this covert drug from our food and drink. In fact, I submit that the primary reason Atkin diets are successful is not so much in the limiting of carbohydrates, but in the fact that people are eliminating the processed foods loaded with this drug that is masquerading as a flavor enhancer! We need to understand the link to this covert drug with ADHD and autism in our kids, and Alzheimer's, ALS (Lou Gehrig's Disease), and Parkinson's disease in our elderly population. But most importantly of all, we need to understand that this drug is in fact **making us obese and diabetic**!

Following the conclusion of WWII, America entered an unprecedented era of materialism and prosperity. Television sets soon became a standard fixture in a typical middle class home. Following the unrest and economic upheavals of the 60's, the majority of the nation's wives and mothers entered the workforce, striving to keep their high standard of living intact while seeking after a professional career of their own. The prototypical home-cooked meal became a rarity with both mom and dad working 9 to 5, or even longer. "Convenient and Fast" became the marketing rally cry. As one famous, feminine T-shirt saucily declared in the 70's, "If you are what you eat, then I am cheap, quick, and easy!"

Soon Madison Avenue and a handful of food manufacturers capitalized on the trend. Processed foods began with the "TV Dinner". Entrepreneurs like Ray Kroc (McDonalds) and Harlan Sanders (Kentucky Fried Chicken) successfully franchised their burger stands and chicken houses from Maine to California – and within a decade additional, rabidly competitive, "fast-food" chains were born. Now, "fast-food" chains are big business, and one of the most competitive of all segments of American capitalism. And why? In 1970, Americans spent a mere $6 billion on "fast-food". It was a multi-billion dollar industry then. In the year 2000, however, Americans spent over $110 billion on "fast-food".[ii]

Every single day that we pick up a magazine, newspaper, or turn on the TV, we are exposed and most definitely influenced by a blitz of advertising exhorting us and our little ones to "consume this, eat there, etc." Little wonder that America's media outlets (TV, magazines, and newspapers) have not exposed the excito-toxin problem. Without a doubt, telling the truth would place their multi-billion dollar advertising revenues at risk, and therefore their businesses. This is another way in which Big Business Buries the Truth!

Multi-national corporations such as Pizza Hut, McDonalds, Burger King, Taco Bell, Coca Cola and Pepsi are now bribing school boards and pubic universities across this country to have their food and drinks exclusively served in the school's cafeterias, lunchrooms, and student commons. Processed snack and convenient fast-foods with low nutritional mineral content and high chemical additive counts are quickly becoming the mainstays and norms of the new millennium. Teens and young adults have grown up with these trends. Who can argue when the food does indeed taste wonderful, and is delivered hot and aromatic within minutes or even seconds? Who can argue when on our high school and college campuses, it is highly "popular" and "vogue" to eat lunch at Burger King or Wendy's instead of packing a lunch from home?

Why does the food taste and smell so very incredible? It's simply because of the special secret ingredient "chemical" additive that when blended and increased in content makes even the cheapest cuts of meat and the blandest of vegetables literally burst with flavors. But Americans need to understand the price we are paying for this burst of flavorful convenience is really much higher than what is posted on the menu boards.

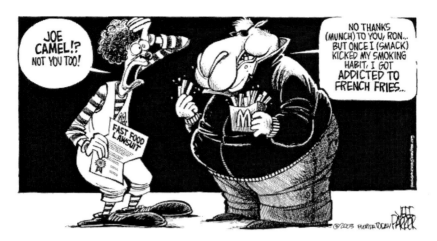

All processed food products and fast food chains have really only one criteria to meet – they have to be so uniquely great tasting that Junior would happily prefer a burger, chicken sandwich, fries, coke, or shake over Mother's meat loaf casserole. They also had to have a "secret sauce" or some secret coating recipe for their deep fried foods that would elevate themselves over their competition in the discerning taste buds of their hungry, yet discriminating public. If a laboratory could produce a substance that really excited the taste buds while producing a very real CRAVING for it, how much PROFIT could be generated by that franchise? Answer: **Big Business Buries the Truth!** Of course, the story line actually begins a few years earlier. Let's take a look at what occurred.

During the occupation of Japan by Allied forces at the conclusion of WWII, the US servicemen noticed something very peculiar. Their Japanese counterparts enjoyed a much tastier chow line. The food was noticeably better tasting than the Allied troop's chipped beef and grits. Why? The resulting Culinary Investigation Team soon found out.

They uncovered that a Japanese biochemist named Dr. Ikeda discovered in 1907 that he could manufacture specific amino acids by means of a process of bacteriological fermentation, replicating a two thousand year old "secret" Japanese process that was used primarily by the Emperor and his elite guard. It was part of the sacred secrets of the Sumo, and was undoubtedly part of the recipe to produce a champion wrestler (food that created large and rapid weight gains while decreasing intellect) – who then gave the glory and honor back to his Lord, the Emperor himself.

Dr. Ikeda patented the unique chemical fermentation process, and then helped to start a company to manufacture and market the end product - monosodium glutamate produced by means of bacteriological fermentation. He named the company Ajinomoto – which literally means in English – "The essence of taste". By the mid 1930's, Ajinomoto's brand of processed glutamic acid was a standard flavor enhancer of Japanese cuisine. It made regular beef, chicken and pork much tastier and more succulent. At least that's what the taste buds report to the brain. The name coined for this wonderful chemical stimulant (i.e. drug) of the taste buds that has so successfully invaded American cuisine?   L-Glutamatic acid monosodium salt, aka Monosodium Glutamate, aka MSG, aka RL-50, aka Accent.

At this point, you are probably saying to yourself – "oh yeah, I've heard of that stuff – that's that mysterious seasoning that's put in Chinese food! I really don't have to worry about that, whenever I eat at my favorite Chinese buffet, I make sure they don't add any to MY plate!" If you are thinking this – please read on. The information you are about to receive may save your life, or at the very least – increase your chances of maintaining at least some semblance of good health well into your 90's.

But is MSG really a drug? It depends on whom you talk to! By it's very definition, a drug is a chemical chain that has been artificially manufactured (and patented) by humans to stimulate or enhance physical or mental processes. MSG, in my opinion, fits this description. Through a patented, proprietary, and totally unnatural fermentation process that UTILIZES CHEMICALLY MUTATED BACTERIA, Ajinomoto's form of MSG is born. There is no doubt about the adverse effect it has on the human brain and the Central Nervous System. This is well documented by Dr. Russell Blaylock in his landmark book. Why then, is it allowed to be added to our food supply? That is the billion-dollar question that the FDA has been ducking for the last two decades. The answer is Big Business Buries the Truth. You need to make up your own mind, however. This may help you. In Ajinomoto's own literature we read how their MSG is produced:

"Since the discovery of Corynebacterium Glutamicum as an efficient Glutamate-overproducing microorganism in 1957, the production of L-amino acids by the fermentative method has become one of the most important research-target of industrial microbiology. Several research groups have developed metabolic engineering principles for L-amino acid-producing C. Glutamicum strains over the last four decades. The mechanism of L-Glutamate-overproduction by the microorganism is very unique and interesting. L. Glutamate overproduction by this bacterium, a

biotin auxotroph, is induced by a biotin limitation and suppressed by an excess of biotin. Addition of a surfactant or penicillin is known to induce L-Glutamate overproduction under excess biotin. After the development of the general molecular biology tools such as cloning vectors and DNA transfer technique, genes encoding biosynthetic enzymes were isolated. With those genes and tools, recombinant DNA technology can be applied in analysis of biosynthetic pathways and strain construction of C. Glutamicum. [xiii]

Unless you are a research biologist, this explanation probably made little or no sense.   Let me interpret it in layman's terms. Corynebaterium Glutamicum (C-Glutamicum) is a genetically modified strain of bacteria, bio-engineered and designed specifically to disintegrate protein molecules of a certain strain of seaweed. This genetically manipulated bacteria does its work in gigantic vats similar to waste water treatment facilities, where the "new form" of monosodium glutamates are subsequently harvested and packaged as MSG.   This is all a process of so-called "recombinant DNA technology" or gene-splicing. To even remotely intimate that MSG as produced by recombinant DNA altered bacteria is a "naturally occurring" substance is simply not accurate. In fact, it is dishonest.

The truth that is hidden by Big Business is that this "Patented Process" produces a form of monosodium glutamate that is unfortunately accompanied by other carcinogenic substances.   L-glutamate is only slightly altered from the naturally occurring glutamate amino acid, but it is altered nevertheless. Here is a simplified explanation of how MSG is produced.

MSG can best be described as "processed free glutamic acid." It is formed when a protein molecule is either fully, or partially broken apart into its basic components, which are individual amino acids. Protein can be broken into its basic amino acids in a number of different ways. In the human gut, various digestive enzymes do the job very effectively. To accomplish the task outside the human gut, chemicals need to be utilized – historically acids and enzymes were utilized, but in the 1950's, Ajinomoto patented the use of specialized bacteria to accomplish it by means of fermentation. The process of isolating "free glutamic acid" is technically referred to as "hydrolyzation of protein" or "hydrolyzed protein", and most papers explaining the process are authored by employees of Ajinomoto, Inc. Therefore, the creation of MSG is somewhat shrouded in mystery, and the Truth is difficult to find. Thanks to brilliant biochemists like Linda K. Hegstrand, the mystery can be solved.

It is interesting to note that the secret to creating large amounts of processed free glutamic acid (MSG) by means of bacterial fermentations is simply not openly discussed by the food manufacturing industry. I believe this is because of the fact that the process perfected by Ajinomoto utilizes genetically engineered (altered) strains of bacteria. Does it not seem a bit strange that when Ajinomoto mentions how their MSG is produced, they talk about it being produced from seaweed, beets, corn, soy, or some other crop, but do not ever describe their use of genetically manipulated bacteria? Is there something distasteful to the general public if they understood the entire process? I believe the answer to that is summed up in one word: Absolutely!!

Different strains of seaweed had been used by oriental cultures to enhance the flavor of foods for thousands of years. Following Dr. Ikeda's discovery in 1907 of glutamic acid, methods for commercially extracting glutamic acid from seaweed were soon developed. From 1910 to 1956, the production of monosodium glutamate was one of chemical extraction, a slow and very costly method. In 1956, with the backing of U.S. chemists and biologists, the Japanese succeeded in mass producing glutamic acid by means of fermentation, and once the bacteria's DNA was altered to increase the yields, the large scale commercial production of monosodium glutamate by means of fermentation began in earnest. The rest is literally history.

Today, the glutamic acid component of monosodium glutamate is produced primarily by means of bacterial fermentation, and the bacteria used are in fact genetically engineered. This little secret is not openly discussed for obvious reasons. To produce MSG by this method, the bio-engineered bacteria are grown and cultured aerobically in a liquid medium containing a source of carbon (typically dextrose or citrate), mineral ions, growth hormone factors, and most importantly, a nitrogen source consisting of ammonium ions in the form of urea. Little wonder this is such a big secret, who would want to consume a product born and processed out of urea? In a nutshell, the bio-engineered bacteria absorb the carbon, growth factors, and nitrate and eventually they excrete the glutamic acid as a "waste product" outside of their cell membrane into the liquid medium (known as 'fermentation broth'). The glutamic acid is then separated from the "broth" by means of filtration, evaporative concentration, acidification, and then crystallization, wherein the final conversion to its monosodium salt form is completed and it is packaged and labeled as monosodium glutamate (MSG).

Following the breakdown of the algae's (or corn, wheat, molasses, etc) protein via the recombinant bacterial fermentation process, some unwanted contaminants unfortunately accompany the MSG. Free glutamic acid (MSG) you see, carries with it material not found with actual, naturally occurring, or unprocessed glutamic acid. Unprocessed glutamic acid is in the form of L-glutamic acid only, while MSG (processed glutamic acid) is both L-glutamic acid and D-glutamic acid, and is also accompanied by pyroglutamic acid and other toxic contaminants. The levels of contaminants differ according to the materials and methods used to produce the glutamic acid – specifically the type and concentration of urea. ***In short, the processed MSG is often accompanied by mono and dichloro propanols (known carcinogens) or heterocyclic amines (which are also highly carcinogenic).***

Here is where the story really gets interesting. By FDA rules and regulations, and by definition, MSG as processed free glutamic acid is classified as "naturally occurring" because the basic ingredient (glutamic acid) is indeed found in nature. Unfortunately for American consumers, "naturally occurring" does not mean that a food additive is being USED in its natural state, or even PRODUCED AND HARVESTED in its natural state! The term "naturally occurring" according to the FDA's infinite wisdom, only means that the food additive BEGAN with something found in nature. By virtue of this FDA "loophole", MSG is classified as organic and natural and can be added to food in any quantity without regulation. I would point out to the FDA that arsenic and lead are also "naturally occurring". So is hydrochloric acid. So is urine or urea. Clearly, "natural" does not necessarily mean "safe"!

You need to also understand that according to the FDA, only when a hydrolyzed protein contains 79% free glutamic acid content or more (the remaining 21% composed of sodium, moisture, and the aforementioned contaminants) is the product required to be labeled as monosodium glutamate, or MSG. When the product contains less than 79% free glutamic acid, the FDA does not require that the ingredients be identified on the label as "containing MSG". This is where the "imposter MSG" labeling is born, with names such as hydrolyzed protein, autolyzed yeast, artificial flavoring, etc. being utilized. This simply means that there is less than 79% free glutamic acid – however, the contaminant level could be higher while the MSG percentage may be as high as 78%. Many people wrongfully think that many of their favorite foods and restaurants are "MSG free", and many fast-food outlets today advertise their entrées "contain no MSG", when in truth however, they utilize 3 or more additives with "less than 79% glutamic acid". It is still MSG folks! Thanks to the FDA rule, these additives are not labeled as MSG, but they still contain potentially damaging amounts of free glutamic acids nevertheless. Often, the combinations of these additives are much more damaging to the body's glutamate receptors than a relatively small amount of pure MSG as listed on the label. So in short, consumers beware!!

As outlined so well by Dr. Blaylock, the processed form of glutamic acid (MSG, hydrolyzed protein, autolyzed yeast, etc.) in even small quantities causes the brain to perceive false signals, hunger sensations are over stimulated, and the body then "craves" foods that include MSG. When this occurs, the body's metabolism slows, and unnatural weight gains are very often the result. In short, it stimulates the human brain and the Central Nervous System into unnatural cravings, often causing addictions. The process is very similar to the effect of nicotine in cigarettes. MSG can well be called the "nicotine of food".

To sum up, the health dangers to humans outlined above are caused by these very subtle ninja assassins in food. These "secret assassins" in turn cause the substance to be "craved" and then over-consumed. What is then consumed is much more quickly and readily absorbed into the blood stream than the truly "natural" or "bound" form of the amino. This combination often causes toxicity and numerous health problems, not the least of which is chronic obesity and a myriad of neurological symptoms. The chemical also causes an increase in the "hunger sensation". Even though sufficient calories have been consumed to satisfy the body's needs, the brain has been fooled into believing there is a caloric deficiency. This is why people often feel ravenously hungry only an hour or so after consuming a large meal of MSG-laden Chinese/Japanese cuisine, or MSG-enhanced fast foods. This is also why our children are becoming obese at a very young age. The MSG they consume in their daily meals makes their bodies store fat in a totally unnatural, very unhealthy way.

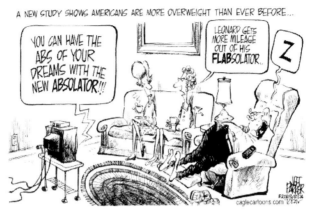

What an incredibly stealthy toxin MSG is! It subtly causes disease symptoms, while it provides its manufacturer with a truly sustainable argument, which is simply that there is no "measurable change" in the naturally occurring glutamic acid. Please do not be fooled. There is indeed a "measurable change", even though it is very subtle indeed. MSG, or L-glutamic acid as it is called in laboratory circles, is in fact produced via specialized bacteria, and is not in reality naturally occurring. It is indeed a Secret Assassin, a Ninja of the Taste Buds!

The incredible truth is that even though the chemical MSG in such excess amounts can, and should be defined as an excito-toxin, it is nevertheless so very pervasive in our American society today that it is EXTREMELY DIFFICULT to avoid. When I discovered the products it has been added to, it occurred to me that there might possibly be a more sinister agenda at work than just increasing corporate profits and bank accounts. Could it be possible that there are individuals in this country who wish to see American brainpower and personal IQ's reduced, and to keep the "silent majority" fat and complacent in order to further some private, corporate agenda? Are certain corporate executives in the food and pharmaceutical industries, (individuals who are extremely well educated in bio-chemistry, extremely wealthy and powerful and who wield incredible influence over our elected politicians), deliberately creating a population that is obese and sickly so we can be more easily dominated and controlled while ever more of their chemical drugs are purchased as a result? Or is it because they are completely innocent and naïve about the excitotoxin dangers they have unwittingly and innocently created, and are only looking at generating ever-increasing profits? I would hope with all of my heart and soul that the MSG and Aspartame poisoning of America is due to nothing more than corporate greed, greed that is only seeking to increase profits in the processed and fast food industries. Such would be merely an "innocent mistake". That is bad enough, if it is not immediately admitted and corrected. To date, however, the problem is barely defined, let alone admitted and corrected. However, after in-depth reading and research, I must declare that I cannot justify any logical reason for MSG being added to yearly Flu shots and MMR vaccines; injections that are given to America's small children before they enter public schools. MSG cannot be added solely to increase vaccination profits, or to "preserve" the pathogens. It is clearly not there to improve the taste, since the vaccines are directly injected. What then is the true agenda?

The German philosopher Goethe eloquently stated many years ago, "No man is more hopelessly enslaved than he who wrongly believes that he is free!" Folks, I would submit that there is no more ponderous ball and chain and more secure slave shackle than a life sentence of diabetes, heart disease, and gross obesity. Furthermore, there is absolutely no doubt that these chronic health challenges are directly linked to MSG and Aspartame. We need to ask ourselves only one question: Who profits? Ultimately, it is the insanely large industrial complex called Pharmacopia, the American Pharmaceutical giants, and giant food processing corporations who are the primary benefactors. It is Pharmacopia that will reap the grisly harvest of highly inflated drug sales from a diseased populace. Yet another example of Big Business Buries the Truth.

Sadly, one of the biggest concerns of America's "Seniors" are the burgeoning costs of prescription drugs whittling away their fixed incomes. This is a very cruel form of inflation, and in my opinion borders on criminal. Many Seniors have become totally dependent on prescription drugs in order to function somewhat "normally". However, being on fixed incomes, they often have to sacrifice other vitally important items to pay for their new prescriptions. Our Seniors surely deserve better in their "Golden Years" don't they?

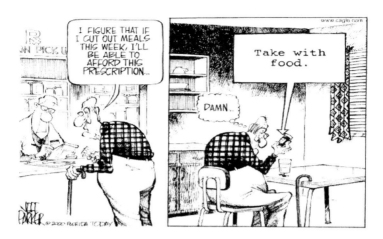

Two very brave doctors, neurosurgeon Russell L. Blaylock, M.D., and emergency room physician George B. Schwartz, M.D. have risked their careers and livelihoods by publishing groundbreaking warnings on MSG, and it's 1st cousin named Aspartame (aka Nutrasweet, Equal). Dr. Blaylock's incredible book *Excitotoxins – the Taste that Kills* leaves little doubt about the biological effects MSG and Aspartame have on the specialized receptors in the human brain and eventually the other organs in the body. Dr. Schwartz's book *In Bad Taste: The MSG Syndrome* likewise systematically outlines the very real dangers posed by this manufactured drug that is now such an intrusive part of American culture.

Thanks to Dr. John W. Olney and Dr. Schwartz's crusade, MSG is no longer added to BABY FOOD. Dr. Olney could not fathom why a supposedly benign taste enhancer like MSG would need to be added to baby foods – after all, a small child really doesn't have a choice in what food they prefer to eat do they? And really, is there anything more primal, yet more wonderfully nourishing than human breast milk from a baby's perspective? Of course not. Then why add MSG to infant "formulas"?

Consequently this brave pioneer blew the whistle loud and hard, testifying before Congress about the MSG dangers. His work paid off with results and it was soon removed voluntarily from baby food (thank God). However, it is still added to certain infant milk formulas, and it remains one of the main ingredients in vaccinations, including flu vaccines as well as hospital IV solutions. WHY IS THIS TRUE, if MSG is truly nothing more than a "flavor enhancer"? Since vaccines do not need to have improved tastes, the only logical conclusion is that if Dr. Blaylock is accurate and MSG is a causative factor in many disease states; adding MSG to vaccines could greatly increase sales of drugs produced by the same companies that manufactured the vaccines containing MSG. The "Problem, Reaction, Solution" scenario is enacted in a very cunning manner. And Big Business Buries the Truth.

MSG entered the American food chain in 1948. Since then, it has been linked to more toxic reactions than almost any other food additive.[iv] Little wonder that certain infants develop brain damage and are diagnosed as autistic after receiving MSG dosages directly into their bloodstream, along with cultures of Mumps, Measles, and Rubella pathogens (MMR Vaccinations). Toxic Mercury is also found in vaccines, but I suspect that MSG may be much more problematic. What happens to every other immunized child that does not become autistic? A few may soon exhibit Attention Deficit Symptoms, but rest assured, ALL who receive MSG directly into their blood as young toddlers (12-18 months of age) will have their endocrine systems, pineal glands, and accompanying neuron receptors permanently affected to some degree.[v]

What exactly is the function of the pineal gland? It is an organ located in the center of the brain that is about the size of a mature pea. It is sensitive to fluctuations in light levels, as perceived through a direct nerve connection to the eyes. Darkness signals the pineal gland to release a hormone called melatonin, which in turn helps the body attain deep, healing REM cycles of sleep. It is during these deep REM cycles of sleep when the human stem cells repair and regenerate cellular damage caused by ageing or injury. Without deep, restful sleep, the body heals much slower and ages much faster.[vi] It is also at a much higher risk to develop chronic, life-threatening diseases.

So, in a very real sense, the pineal gland acts very much like the control desk and dispatcher for 911 emergency calls. The pineal gland works in harmony with the hypothalamus gland, directing the body's thirst, hunger, sexual drive and desire, and is the biological clock that determines our aging process. It is the "third eye" of the brain, responsible for telling the brain when it is day or night. It also controls the body's hormonal systems, sleep-wake cycle, and other so-called "circadian" (24-hour) body rhythms. It is in essence, the body's internal clock. In short, it is one of the most important organs in the human body.

Recent research has uncovered even more startling facts. This amazing little pea-sized organ is also the intuitive and cognitive reasoning center of the human endocrine system. The pineal gland's chemical secretions help to instill individuality and creativity, regulating and providing euphoric emotions, relieves stress and anxiety and is responsible for inter-dimensional spiritual connections that often occurs during deep REM sleep cycles.[vii] It is, in a nutshell, the essence of the human soul. To the ancient Greeks, it was literally referred to as the "Seat of the Soul", a theory reaffirmed by the French physiologist and mathematician Descartes, in the early 1600's. However, the biological role of the pineal gland was not clearly established until 1958. When humans are under increased stress, the pineal gland produces much less melatonin, resulting in "sleepless nights" and eventually, disease states. The role of the pineal gland and melatonin in health and healing is extremely vital to understand.

To me, the pineal gland is much more than the seat of good health. It is clearly the seat of genius as well. It kindles the fires of passion and desires for individual freedom and expression. It is undeniable that an adult with restricted or damaged pineal gland neurons is more likely willing to "conform" and not seek new information nor question the status quo. They undoubtedly become more subservient to authority figures, and tend to trust government bureaucracies completely. They show less emotion. In short, they make great slaves, because they have lost the ability to DREAM. Is it just a coincidence that school districts across America have made it a basic requirement to have their pupils uniformly vaccinated with serums laced with MSG excitotoxins that in turn attack the pineal gland neurons before they can get an "education" as prescribed by a

"Board of Regents" thereby becoming "model citizens"?   And we think Orwell's '1984' is merely a work of fiction?

Once again to sum up, MSG is a basic amino acid that is produced via a fermentation process utilizing DNA manipulated bacteria. Amino Acids are the basic building blocks of proteins that are found in all living things. Nutritional scientists have identified 20 different types of amino acids used by the human body. Our brain and many major organs in our body use the Glutamate amino acid. MSG in natural or "bound" state is a vital nutrient, but when in a "freed state" the blood absorbs the amino acid 8-10 times faster than normal and the neurons in the brain are subsequently damaged. Regardless of the endless propaganda spewed by MSG manufactures to the contrary, MSG is NOT a completely natural substance, and it is most definitely NOT healthy to consume. Otherwise, it would not kill mice and rats in laboratory testing. The Big Business interests are burying the truth by wanting biochemists to believe and teach the masses that MSG is dangerous only in very large amounts, because after all it is a natural form of glutamine (False).

This propaganda is like saying that a single harmless carbon atom that is bound to a single, harmless oxygen molecule forms a totally natural and harmless new gas, because its individual molecular components are totally benign and harmless. But everyone (especially those who are contemplating a painless suicide) knows that CO (carbon monoxide) is an odorless, colorless, tasteless gas that kills very efficiently after only a few deep breaths, because it very quickly robs the blood of essential oxygen molecules. Add just one more "totally benign and harmless oxygen molecule" to CO and you have CO_2, (carbon dioxide) which is not nearly as toxic when inhaled. (But when it is added to water to form fizzy soda pop, it too robs oxygen from the brain much like CO does, only it does it much slower!) Another example is propyl alcohol and iso-proplyl alcohol. Both substances have the exact number of atoms in its structure, but they are structurally different, and therefore have different names and different chemical activities. Add just one more hydrogen molecule, plus a charged sodium ion to glutamine and it changes its structure and function as well.

The difference between mineral elements such as gold and iridium and lead is just a couple of small, "insignificant" electrons in the shell and a matching proton. That's it – that's all it takes. Were not even talking about another complete molecule, just a couple of electrons and matching protons! Is gold the same as lead and iridium? Of course not, they are as different as night and day. Their molecular weight and individual vibratory frequencies are much different. They are therefore different elements with different characteristics. Furthermore, gold and iridium mineral elements have health-promoting energies, while lead is toxic. The only differences between these elements are a few seemingly insignificant electrons. The same is true with MSG – it is most definitely not a naturally occurring glutamine amino acid. Because of the medium in which it is born, it has more potential contaminants than naturally occurring glutamic amino acids, and is much more readily absorbed into the blood stream! As long as officials at the FDA keep buying into Ajinomoto's propaganda and half-truths, meaningful warnings and regulations will be very slow in coming.

Unlike most chemical additives that we consume, MSG has been proven to pass very quickly into the bloodstream and can enter the brain and organs directly. Once inside the brain and organs, it causes the nerve endings in the brain and organs (called neurons) to fire uncontrollably. The brain gets a very confused signal from the neuron sensors. It translates this over-stimulation of the nerves to be perceived as good taste and increased flavor. Furthermore, when a neuron is "over-stimulated", it eventually dies. In the over-stimulated neuron's last few hours of life, it fires signals away uncontrollably, sending the electrical excitement induced by the MSG amino to the cognitive portion of our brain. Anywhere from two to twenty-four hours later, the neuron is dead, and its neural pathways where your thoughts and cognitive reasoning travel is terminated. The mental pathway it had once bridged to the Central Nervous System and the brain has been permanently destroyed.

The process of destruction of brain neurons by MSG and Aspartame is very similar to placing too high of an electrical voltage on a computer's motherboard, typical in the case of a "power surge". The pathways the electrical impulses usually travel are "over-excited" by too much electrical energy, becomes short-circuited, and your computer no longer works. It has to have either a major repair, or it has to be replaced.

It must be pointed out that MSG does not affect everyone in the same way, however. For instance, some people have stronger, healthier cells thanks to specific genetic markers that produce more cellular energy (ATP) than others. Some people have had head injuries that have already damaged a large number of neurons, and MSG affects them much more powerfully. Others have genetic weaknesses in their cellular DNA allowing them to be highly sensitive to the MSG compound. It is estimated that 40% of all people are "highly sensitive" to MSG's toxicity, however, and this number is growing every year.[viii]

Unfortunately, without proper mineral nutrition, the brain has difficulty creating new neurons, and is forced instead to relearn and re-program new neural pathways around the damaged areas. A by-product of this is lower I.Q. and much lower cognitive reasoning skills, chronic headaches, and irritability. The brain cells and the neuron pathways where they function that you are born with are designed to last a lifetime. In just a few short hours, MSG has literally excited many of your brain cells to death. This is why MSG is rightly named an "excito-toxin".[ix]

Fortunately for us, the human brain contains approximately ten trillion neurons, and each neuron supports up to 10,000 individual pathways. Clearly, the most sophisticated computer system on earth literally pales in comparison to the intricacies and complexities of the human brain. Because of this complexity, MSG and Aspartame's toxic effects do not kill or maim immediately. It happens slowly over time, and the symptoms appear very subtly. As one group of neurons perish, others may take their place if you consume correct minerals and other healthy nutritional building blocks. But inevitably, damage does occur. Depending on your genetic tendencies, you may not become totally, or even partially debilitated. Then again, however, you may well "come down" with Alzheimer's, Parkinson's disease, diabetes, or some other disease state, and when you do, your quality of life becomes greatly reduced. Is it worth the risk? I would submit, the ravages of ageing are bad enough without helping it along by unwittingly consuming excito-toxins. Perhaps more troublesome is the effect MSG and Aspartame is having on future generations. Often, toxic brain cell alterations are more noticeable in the 2nd or 3rd generations.

I remember a TV commercial a decade or so ago. It showed a picture of an egg being your brain. When the egg was heated and began to sizzle, the caption read- this is your brain on drugs. The sizzling effects of excito-toxins on the brain as described by Dr. Blaylock, remind me of that advertisement. Americans are frying their brains unwittingly. Have you ever heard of children today, especially those with ADHD diagnosis, being referred to as "over-stimulated"?

When the brain perceives food to taste incredibly good, our central nervous system tells our body to consume more and more of it. A typical situation is when one cracks open a fresh bag of MSG laden potato chips, or a bag of goldfish crackers. Who can just eat one handful? Often, Americans continue "snacking" on such products even after the hunger sensation is well satisfied. How often have you opened a bag or box of such snacks, only to discover mere minutes later that it was empty? How often have you done this without any family member present – in other words, how often have you downed the whole bag all by yourself? Such "binging" is especially dangerous, as it tends to elevate the blood Glutamate to potentially toxic levels.

We wonder, (as I did for over 10 years) why it is that a record number of adults as well as children have been diagnosed as being obese in today's Western society. There is not much doubt in my mind that MSG consumption has made it much easier to put on the extra pounds.

Again, please note that in literally hundreds of studies published in North America and abroad, researchers routinely administer MSG to newborn mice and rats to induce highly abnormal obesity within days of birth. Next the researchers use the MSG-injected, obese rodents for research on such diseases as diabetes and, sickeningly, weight loss MEDICATIONS!! Instead of enlisting advertising executives to brainwash the public into buying their weight-loss drugs tested on MSG-induced obese rats and mice, why not educate the American masses that the single most important step to losing weight healthily and naturally involves limiting their intake of MSG "free-Glutamates"?! Because Big Business Buries the Truth!

Incredibly, according to Drs. Olney and Blaylock, humans develop higher blood levels of free glutamate excitotoxins following ingestion of MSG than does any other animal species tested. [x] Dr. Olney notes that: "The amount of MSG in a single bowl of commercially available soup is probably enough to cause blood glutamate levels that predictably cause brain damage in immature animals."[xi]

Dr. Olney found that human children are often exposed to acute MSG intakes in the range of 100 to 150 mg/kg only by consuming processed manufactured foods. In humans tested, this amount (100-150 mg/kg) caused a twenty-fold elevation in their blood glutamate levels. In comparison, mice ingesting the same amount develop only a four-fold increase in blood glutamate levels.[xii] Remember that most of the initial research that has shown glutamate to be destructive to the brain was done using mice. Studies now show that humans absorb 5 TIMES MORE glutamate into the blood than mice, and Dr. Olney tells us that the amount of MSG in a single bowl of MSG-enhanced commercially produced soup "predictably causes brain damage" in infant mice. Wow! Even more alarming is what the pharmaceutical giant Merck tells us about MSG. The median lethal dose, or the quantity of a chemical that is estimated to be fatal to 50% of the organisms tested (LD50) for MSG is only 19.9 grams per kilogram of body weight when ingested gastro-intestinally.[xiii] If Dr. Olney's calculations are accurate, then the median lethal dosage for humans is around 6-8 ounces, depending on your weight. While it may be true that nobody is going to accidentally ingest 6-8 ounces of Accent™ MSG seasoning, there is little doubt that the toxic effects of this covert drug accumulate over time. It can only best be described as a "Secret Assassin". According to researcher Dr. Adrienne Samuels, Americans consumed 12 grams of MSG per person per year in 1960. In 2000, Americans consumed in excess of 500 grams/person/year. It is truly a miracle and a testament of the adaptability of the human body that we are not all brain dead. On second thought, perhaps we are, or we wouldn't be consuming nearly so much of an excitotoxic poison.

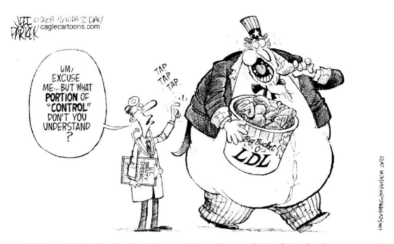

I thought initially that I could make a list of typical grocery items that had MSG included in its ingredients chart to publish in this book. But after a trip to my local grocery store, I soon realized that I did not have enough space in the book to list all the products. Over 200 items had MSG in at least one form or another, and I had only made it down two aisles. I was totally and completely shocked and more than a little stunned. I had no idea the problem was this big. No wonder America is largely sick, I told myself. How dreadful! Without a doubt, our government allows Big Business to Bury the Truth. How sad this truth is – because it is in reality so very unnecessary.

Here is just a small sampling of foods that contain MSG:

Bouillon Cubes	Pasta Helpers	Flavored Rice
Soy Sauce	Ice Cream	Sour Cream
Seasoning Mixes	Cheese Puffs	Jerky
Frozen Entries	Gravy	Frozen Diet Entrees
Salad Dressings	Frozen Cured Meat	Frozen Potatoes
Vegetable Juice	Dried Soup Mix	Canned Meats

Canned Pastas	Canned Chili	Ramen Noodles (Major Source)
Wieners	Bologna	Canned Soups (Major Source)
Potato Chips	Nachos	Flavored Crackers
Gelatin Desserts	Fruit Drinks (Watch out for "Flavor Enhancers")	

Keep in mind, that often MSG is hidden in other ingredients on the la

bel. I will discuss this in greater detail later in the book, but if the label shows it has gelatin, autolyzed yeast, yeast extract, hydrolyzed plant or animal protein, and "natural" or "artificial" flavoring then please understand, it has MSG. Worse, many items have 2, 3, 4 or more combinations of MSG ingredients in it. One product I saw listed: Monosodium Glutamate, Hydrolyzed Animal Protein, Yeast extract, Natural Flavorings, and Autolyzed Yeast on its label. Historically, this particular barbecued potato chip product had been one of my favorite foods. No wonder I mysteriously gained weight, and had common migraine headaches, even though I exercise and eat sensibly otherwise (as far as volumes are concerned).

If you are really serious about improving your life, losing weight naturally, and truly care about protecting your loved ones from a life sentence of debilitating chronic illness – you need to do your best to eliminate MSG (and its 1st cousin Aspartame) as much as possible from your diet. But understand, that is much easier said than done. It is going to take a lot of sacrifice. You see, virtually all snack foods, refined foods, prepared frozen entrees and processed meats for sale in the U.S. have more than two MSG-rich ingredients added. Soups are literally loaded with MSG, especially the Top Ramen style soups which have levels as high as 40% MSG in their powdered base. This is especially dangerous because MSG in liquid form raises the free l-glutamate levels in the blood much faster than in its dried or powdered form.

Just for kicks, I visited restaurants and fast-food chains in the Salt Lake City area, and asked them for a complete list of ingredients that are added to their most popular menu items. Almost without exception, I was referred to the manager, who looked at me like I had just arrived from Mars. After telling them I was doing a research project on food-borne allergies, I usually received the detailed ingredient lists. The majority of the managers told me that their meat products contained "absolutely no" MSG. It wasn't that they were lying to me, it was just that they truly didn't know or understand that monosodium glutamate, or hydrolyzed protein was MSG. I found the following chains serve foods laced with MSG, and I am extremely confident that many others do as well. I don't wish to single out just these few, for my list is far from exhaustive. Don't be shy about asking to see a restaurant's ingredients list – as this is now required by law in most states. The restaurants serving up MSG in their menu items include (but is not limited to): A&W, Applebee's, Arby's, Boston Market, Burger King, Carl's Jr. Chili's, Cracker Barrel, Dairy Queen, Denny's, Domino's Pizza, Golden Corral, Hard Rock Café, Hardee's, Hooters, IHOP (International House of Pancakes), Jack in the Box, Kentucky Fried Chicken, Long John Silvers, McDonalds, Outback Steakhouse, Pizza Hut, Red Lobster, Ruby Tuesday, Sizzler, Sonic Drive-In, Taco Bell, T.G.I. Friday's, Village Inn, and Wendy's. Keep in mind that I did not analyze all menu items. There may well be some items at these restaurants that are 100% MSG free. You can't be sure, unless you ask, however. If your favorite restaurant cannot provide a complete ingredients list of their most popular menu items, then move on to another one. Don't forget that salad bars are usually a safe bet, but stay away from dressings especially the low-cal, low-fat ones. All dressings are typically loaded with MSG, and you will probably never know it unless you have read this book.

CONCLUSIONS:

The three-pound chemical manufacturing plant called the human brain is a truly amazing and wondrous creation. The repertoire of its chemical actions and reactions are amazingly complex and science has only recently begun to unlock all of its secrets.

Thanks to brilliant neurosurgeons like Dr. Russell Blaylock, the correct and vital role of mineral nutrients in healthy brain functions is becoming better understood. With that understanding also comes the realization of the dangers of certain man-manipulated amino acids such as MSG and Aspartame. It is quite well understood now for instance, that clinical depression's root cause is the lack of electron generation and flow by means of brain chemical imbalances. In turn, low electron flow is caused by a combination of low mineral nutrients and the breakdown of the pineal gland neural pathways, which decreases the secretion and regulation of vital hormones throughout the brain. Dr. Blaylock shows that the malfunction of the pineal gland is largely due to the constant consumption of large amounts of chemical "free glutamates" added to processed foods as MSG.

In understanding the vital need to limit free glutamates while increasing prime mineral nutrients, Dr. Blaylock may have said it best in his book. He declares: "The series of chemical reactions needed to break down glucose in the brain also depends on an adequate supply of minerals and trace elements being present. These act as co-factors and co-enzymes (helpers) that help spur these reactions along. These vital supplements should be supplied, because when deficient, serious disease can occur. Far too many physicians, because of a neglect of nutritional courses in medical training, do not appreciate the critical nature of these nutrients in human health."[xiv]

Later in this book, I will give you specific ideas of which mineral nutrients, and in which correct form, will help the brain neutralize the chemically altered amino acids, the excess excitatory amino acid neurotransmitters called MSG and Aspartame, that may help you regain, or better yet – MAINTAIN, your youthful health and vitality.

---

[i] Neiuwenhuys, R. *Chemoarchitecture of the Brain*, New York: Springer-Verlag, 1988
[ii] Sclosser, Eric. Fast Food Nation, Houghton Miflin, 2001, page 3
[iii] Kimura, E. Fermentation & Biotechnology Laboratories, Ajinomoto Co., Inc.. "Metabolic engineering of Glutamate production." Adv Biochem Eng Biotechnologies 2003; 79:37-57
[iv] Erb, John E. & T. Michelle, The Slow Poisoning of America, Palladins Press, 2003, page 42
[v] Choi, D.E. "Glutamate Neurotoxicity and Diseases of the Nervous System.: *Neuron 1*(1988): 623-634
This excellent article covers all aspects of glutamate toxicity, and shows that even a single dose causes damage to neurons and the endocrine system.
[vi] The Amazing Machine Time Life Books, pp 84-86
[vii] Ibid
[viii] Olney, J.W. "Excitotoxic Food Additives: Functional Teratological Aspects." Prog. Brain Review, 83
[ix] Blaylock, Dr. Russell, Excitotoxins:The Taste that Kills, Health Press, Santa Fe, 1997. Page 42
[x] Ibid: Page 37.
[xi] Olney, J.W. "Excitotoxic Food Additives: Functional Teratological Aspects." Prog. Brain Review, 283-294.
[xii] Ibid. page 296
[xiii] Merck Index, 13th Edition, 2001 – *Merck Research Laboratories* pg. 1117
[xiv] Blaylock, Dr. Russell, Excitotoxins:The Taste that Kills, Health Press, Santa Fe, 1997. Page 23

Chapter 2

The Evidence Accumulates

The dissenter is every human being at those moments of his life when he resigns momentarily from the herd and thinks for himself.
- Archibald MacLeish

All great truths begin as blasphemies.
- George Bernard Shaw

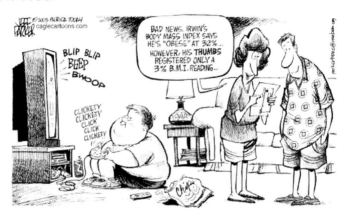

Jane is a typical American mother of four beautiful children – two boys and two girls. She is well educated, having finished her master's degree. She is happy, but she is also concerned. Now that she is over forty, it is virtually impossible for her to maintain that cute, girlish figure that she really began to lose about a decade ago after the birth of her last daughter. What is frustrating Jane the most, however, is that she is constantly counting calories and visits her local health club religiously every morning. She sweats profusely in her aerobics class, and she logs at least 20 miles a week on that stationary bike. What gives? She just can't seem to lose that stubborn 30 pounds she gained since her hysterectomy. But at least she is not like her best friend Betty, who has ballooned up to over 200 pounds. Jane knows that Betty doesn't eat much more than she does, but Betty you see, is just plain lazy – and doesn't want to take the time to exercise. They both have been on the Atkin's low Carb diet for the past year, but a couple of cookies and potato chips meant for their kids always seems to grab them when they pass by their pantries.

Jane consults with her Doctor, and she tells her that she is actually doing very well. Her gynecologist explains that following the onset of menopause, and with the surgical removal of her ovaries, it is totally natural for her body to gain a few extra pounds – but the important thing is to keep the weight somewhat under control. In other words, Jane tells herself, – do not let yourself get like Betty!!

Betty is also a typical American mother. Unlike her neighbor and best friend Jane, however, she has always been a little on the "heavy" side. Her mother and grandmother were both large women, and genetically "heavy boned". But they were never as overweight as Betty has become by her 45th birthday. Jane, while being a good friend, has hurt Betty with a few of her comments on her weight. Betty understands that Jane is only trying to help her, but nevertheless her comments on "lack of motivation" to workout at the gym have left Betty feeling depressed and blue on a number of occasions. Jane just simply doesn't understand her, even though she is her best friend.

Betty's 14-year-old daughter has been taking Ritalin since she was diagnosed at seven with ADHD, and now her two sons are exhibiting signs of teen-age depression and ADHD as well. Betty is exhausted after working part time at the school cafeteria, and meeting with school counselors in the afternoon. It seems at least one of her kids is constantly into some kind of problem every week. Worse, last week the school counselor reported that her daughter confided to one of her friends that she is contemplating suicide. There just seems to be something emotionally comforting about food when she is upset and worried about her children.

Betty keeps telling Jane that she will go to the Gym with her next week, but the energy level today is simply not there. Betty is not lazy, she is just physically and emotionally tired ALL OF THE TIME. Her husband has lost all interest in sex, and seems to be only interested in watching his ball games in the family room. It seems they are only staying married because of the kids.

Betty in reality has worked harder to keep her weight under control than Jane. You see, Betty has only consumed "low-fat entrees" for the last 8 years, and eats a lot of salads with low-cal dressing. She has noticed that it seems strange that she seems to really gain weight soon after receiving her yearly flu shots, but believes that is just a coincidence.

Can you relate to Jane or Betty? Moreover, do you, or anyone you know regularly suffer from the following symptoms to the point of seeking medical help: 1. Severe headaches 2. Irregular heartbeat, or racing heart 3. Depression or mood changes, bipolar, seasonal affective disorders (SAD) 4. Abdominal pain, chronic diarrhea, colitis, nausea 5. Balance problems, dizziness, seizures or mini-strokes 6. Sleep Disorders such as insomnia and daytime sleepiness 7. Tenderness in localized areas, neck, back, shoulders, etc. 8. Intermittent swelling and water gains in hands, feet, legs, and jaw 9. Difficulty in swallowing and gagging reflex 10. Hyperactivity, behavioral problems, difficulty concentrating, poor memory 11. Pain in joints or bones 12. Heavy, weak feeling in arms and legs, restless leg syndrome 13. ADD, ADHD, Rage Disorder 14. Chronic Post Nasal Drip. These are all typical symptoms associated with MSG (D-Glutamate) sensitivity.

Does the following scenario play itself out more often than not in homes across America? Does it happen in yours? If so, you are more than likely a victim of a Secret Assassin, the Ninja of Taste.

It's Saturday afternoon, and the kids have all left with friends. You have procrastinated that health club workout for the past month, and now it's a great time to go. You know that you have gained 6 inches around your middle over the last year, and yet it doesn't seem that you have really indulged in too much "junk food". In fact, just today you proudly congratulated yourself by refusing to sample even a single French Fry from your daughter's Happy Meal, even though they smelled SO GOOD that you almost drooled. All you had was a small order of Chicken Nuggets – and while your stomach is continuously growling, you are still PROUD of yourself. You'll just grab a quick salad then head for the gym.

But wait, you are suddenly drained of energy, and you feel a bit light-headed. Why? All you had was a green salad with some of that tasty low-cal dressing. You tell yourself that you'll feel better after a little 30-minute siesta – then you can hit the gym, right?

After an hour and half nap, you don your workout clothes and head out for the gym. But before you get in your car, you realize now you are hungry again. In fact, you are so hungry that you are now even more dizzy and lightheaded. You tell yourself you had better not drive until you get something in your tummy.

You see, what has happened is the insulin in your blood has increased thanks to the excessive amounts of MSG in your tasty low-fat, low-cal dressing you consumed for lunch. The increased insulin has stripped your body of all excess sugar – and now you are a little weak and light-headed and craving something sweet. "No, I can't have any sugar" you tell yourself, so you take a quick break and grab that box of "healthy low-fat" snack crackers made of partially hydrogenated vegetable proteins and MSG based caseinate to tide you over until after your workout.

Before you know it, however, the cracker box is empty – and it is an hour later. Wow, those crackers really tasted great – you can't believe you ate the whole box – but you tell yourself that the actual reason is because of the fact that even though the cost of the crackers has increased, the volume of product per box has decreased. No wonder the box is empty you tell yourself, because it seems you only had a couple of handfuls.

It's much too late for that health club workout now – besides, the kids will soon be home and they will surely be hungry. No problem, you planned the week's menu out, and all you have to do is crack open that can of teriyaki chicken and steam some rice – and presto, dinner is served. Meanwhile, as you prepare your family's meal, the MSG from the crackers is now coursing through your veins, this time attaching itself to carbohydrate molecules that naturally store themselves away in your thighs, buttocks and waist. You just had a nice long nap, but you just can't figure out why you still feel so drained.   It must be the fact that you are getting older you tell yourself.

In comes the family, and just in time. Your quick and easy stir-fry chicken teriyaki dinner is hot off the stove. Wow, doesn't that dinner smell fabulous – and by golly, it tastes even better!! You watch your family gobble it right up, and you feel great. Such a low-fat dinner – and you are such a fantastic mother – feeling securely warm and fuzzy that your family is eating so healthily. Little do you know that you have just loaded your family up with a large amount of a very potentially dangerous drug called MSG.

You need to understand that it is the fat molecules in food that gives it flavor. When a food is processed to remove fat molecules, making it low-fat, it also becomes low-flavor. American kids (as well as their moms) do not like low flavor products. They will usually only buy them once. Then sales and corporate profits plummet. So savvy manufactures pile on the MSG – the "Essence of Taste", as well as dozens of other "flavor enhancers" that also incorporate MSG in their manufacturing. And all is well. Thanks to the FDA, THERE ARE NO LIMITS TO THE AMOUNT OF MSG THAT CAN BE ADDED TO YOUR FOOD!!

Your low-fat chicken teriyaki dish typically has over 5 MSG enhanced ingredients – including (if you read your label) Monosodium

Glutamate (MSG), Hydrolyzed Plant Protein (fancy name for MSG), Autolyzed Yeast Extract (more MSG), Sodium Caseinate (a fancier name for MSG), and Soy Sauce (yet another source of MSG). But you are an even smarter mom. You made up a wondrously colorful Jello gelatin desert (MSG packed). Low-fat jello to boot (higher MSG). And you topped it with oodles of low-fat non-dairy whipped topping (Even more MSG). Mom, do you know you just dosed your family with 7 large portions of potentially toxic MSG IN THIS ONE MEAL? You have wondered why it is your kids are getting a little plump lately, and have little or no desire to go outside and play. Where is the lure of the outdoors that you had when you were a child? Oh yeah, you tell yourself: "I almost forgot, I didn't have Nintendo Game Cubes when I was a child —and most definitely did not have 300+ cable tv channels to choose from. Of course, how silly of me." No mother, the reality is that most of the children's obesity has been chemically induced by hidden Secret Assassins in the food they consume.

Sunday morning arrives, you crawl out of bed with a dull headache. You slowly make your way into the bathroom, and after relieving yourself you step on the bathroom scales and discover to your shock and amazement that you have gained a full pound. Impossible. All you had all day yesterday was a few crackers, a salad, a small helping of low-fat stir-fry chicken teriyaki over rice, and a small bowlful of low-fat Jello gelatin. Yesterday, you were hungry all day long. Today you feel like the StaPuf Marshmallow Woman. What gives?

Then you tell yourself that there is no chance for you to lose any weight – your metabolism has simply hit the middle-age spread and there is NOTHING you can do about it!   You are going to get fat anyway, so why not enjoy it. It has to be due to all the stress you are under with your work and keeping the house straight! You know it is, because you have a continuous "dull headache" that only leaves you after taking an Advil or two. When you asked him, your family Doctor told you it was "stress-related" and not to worry about it. So today you feel sorry for yourself. To lift your depression, you indulge yourself and bring in the really big guns – a double walnut brownie smothered with Rocky Road ice cream. (If only you knew how much MSG based flavor enhancers went into that carton of ice cream!!) Later on, you are side-lined by a blinding migraine headache. It is tough to fight the full-blown depression that is setting in. You are not happy with your life. If only you were 18 again---------!

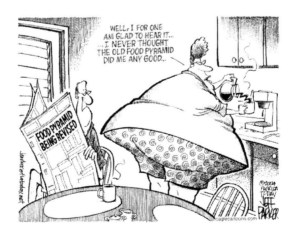

You, along with Jane, Betty, and millions of other Americans, both female and male, need to understand that your weight problem, stress headaches, and other symptoms may not be your fault, or age-related at all. You need to understand how certain chemical drugs added to your food cause you to gain weight while you sleep. You need to understand its profound effect on your metabolism and neurological system. To do this, you need to understand how a pharmaceutical research laboratory produces an obese mouse.

There is simply no such thing as a naturally obese mouse. A mouse needs to be slim and flexible in order to travel efficiently in the small cracks and crevices where it lives and calls home. An obese mouse is unable to survive too long in its natural environment. So, nature has provided the mouse a unique metabolism with glutamate and lepton receptors that very efficiently regulate its fat cells. A mouse can typically eat twice its weight in natural foods such as grain, but will not normally become obese. After a large meal, its metabolism increases, and its fecal droppings increase in volume, but it does not become obese. Also, mice are used in research labs because their organ systems and mammalian genetics are very similar to humans – in other words, what causes reactions in mice will also cause similar reactions in humans at very precise and very predictable ratios.

To effectively test weight-loss drugs and procedures, (thanks in no small part to MSG, weight-loss is now a trillion dollar industry) the research labs have a dilemma. They need to produce obese mice. And how does a lab produce obese mice? They inject them just under the skin with MSG. That's right, the exact same Secret

Assassin chemical that is added to America's food by the ton. And when the testing is complete, how does the same lab euthanize the mice? By injecting a larger amount of pure MSG into the mice's bloodstream of course. This causes the brain to die, while keeping other organs intact for further testing. You see, in large doses, MSG is as deadly as strychnine, but for some reason is not nearly as heavily regulated. Maybe it has to do with corporate profiteering!

For some reason, the FDA has crossed their wires concerning MSG.   On one hand, thanks to some very large political heavyweights, MSG has been given the Generally Recognized As Safe (GRAS) rating – which allows manufacturers to add any amount they want to their food products. On the other hand, the FDA is fully aware that MSG in foods is not as safe as they (and Ajinomoto Inc.) would want you to believe.

The FDA issued a report dated August 31, 1995 that states: "**_Studies have shown that the body uses Glutamate, an amino acid, as a nerve impulse transmitter in the brain and that there are Glutamate-responsive tissues in other parts of the body, as well. Abnormal function of these Glutamate receptors has been linked with certain neurological diseases, such as Alzheimer's disease and Huntington's Chorea. Injections of Glutamate in laboratory animals have resulted in damage to nerve cells in the brain._**"

The report also declares that between 1980 and 1994, there were 622 reports of complaints about side effects from MSG. Additionally, the report shows that in 1992, the FDA asked the Federation of American Societies for Experimental Biology (FASEB) to review all available data on L-Glutamate, (MSG) and present a report on their findings. In the resulting 350 page report, the FASEB concluded specifically that an: *"**Unknown percentage of the population may react to MSG and develop MSG Symptom Complex, a condition characterized by one or more of the following symptoms:**"*

- ➢ *Burning sensation in the back of the neck, forearms, and chest*
- ➢ *Numbness in the back of the neck, radiating to the arms and back*
- ➢ *Tingling, warmth and weakness in the face, temples, upper back, neck, and arms*
- ➢ *Facial pressure or tightness*
- ➢ *Chest Pain*
- ➢ *Headache (including Migraine)*
- ➢ *Nausea*
- ➢ *Rapid Heartbeat (Tachycardia)*
- ➢ *Bronchospasm (difficulty breathing) in MSG-intolerant people with asthma*
- ➢ *Drowsiness*
- ➢ *Weakness*

In otherwise healthy MSG-intolerant people, the MSG Symptoms Complex tends to occur within one hour after eating 3 grams or more of MSG on an empty stomach or without other food. A typical serving of Glutamate-treated food contains less than 0.5 grams of MSG. A reaction is most likely if the MSG is eaten in a large quantity or in a liquid, such as a clear soup."

The FASEB report is remarkable for a couple of reasons. First, it clearly delineates to the FDA that Ajinomoto Inc.'s MSG is most definitely not benign. Bronchospasm is very often deadly to asthmatics, even with a dilator. It also states that there is now a new disease to diagnose: MSG Symptoms Complex, or MSGSC. Also keep in mind that 3 grams is approximately only about ½ of a teaspoon. I am confident that food suppliers put much more than that on a typical entrée, and because of its GRAS rating, there is no limit to the 'Essence of Taste' that can be added. Remember, the more that is added, the better the taste, the more addicting it becomes, and higher profits are generated.

The report also recognizes that a negative reaction is more likely if the MSG is consumed in a liquid soup. All dried soups and Top Ramen products have well over .5 grams of MSG, as do almost all Campbells and Knorr soups. So why is the FDA NOT RESTRICTING IT?

I'll go into this in more detail later on, but what would happen if .5 mgs of pure MSG were inhaled directly into the nasal passages, bypassing the blood-brain barrier and going directly into the brain itself? By their own report's admission, the FDA recognizes that Glutamate injections in lab animals damaged the brain's nerve cells. Surely, therefore, the FDA would never approve a product that allows MSG to be directly inhaled into the olfactory nerves, WOULD THEY??? Sorry, but they have – it's called Flu-Mist produced by Wyeth Inc. (Formerly American Home Products, maker of Fen-Phen).

In his incredible book, Dr. Blaylock exposes the many ways MSG is hidden on food labeling. He has graciously allowed others to quote and draw from his work. If you are serious about losing weight and avoiding becoming a statistic, you MUST LEARN TO READ LABELS and eliminate MSG as completely as possible from your diet. Can losing that extra 30-50 pounds (and keeping it off) possibly be as simple as eliminating MSG from your diet? Yes it may well be, but don't be fooled – it may sound like a simple enough task, but it definitely is not easy to do. Like any other CNS stimulating drug such as nicotine or cocaine, once you begin to restrict it, the body experiences very real "withdrawal symptoms".   Expect a dull headache, irritability, brain fog, and low energy levels for at least two to three weeks while the body releases from its drug-induced stupor. But rest assured, the end result is most definitely worth it – your mind and body can indeed be free!

NOTES

Label Ingredients that ALWAYS contain MSG:

Monosodium Glutamate	Yeast Extract
Monopotassium Glutamate	Glutamic Acid
Hydrolyzed Protein (any and all)	Sodium Caseinate
Yeast Food	Hydrolyzed Corn Gluten
Gelatin (yes, even Jello)	Textured Protein
Yeast Nutrient	Autolyzed Yeast

Ingredients that often contain MSG, or create it during processing:

Carrageenan	Natural Pork Flavoring
Citric Acid	Natural Beef Flavoring
Bouillon and Broth	Natural Chicken Flavoring
Maltodextrin	Whey Protein Concentrate
Soup Stocks	Whey Protein
Ultra Pasteurized	Soy Sauce
Barley Malt	Enzyme (or Enzyme Modified)
Pectin	Malt Flavoring
Protease	Soy Protein
Protease Enzymes	Soy Protein Concentrate
Soy Protein Isolate	Malt Extract

Any Ingredient Labeled 'Fermented' and/or 'Protein Fortified'

AND MOST IMPORTANT – 'NATURAL FLAVORS & SEASONINGS' which is very often a catch-all for MSG based food enhancing ingredients, especially in condiments, spices and salt products.

Keep in mind that certain yeast products like Brewer's Yeast is markedly different than 'autolyzed yeast' and are very healthy to consume, as are certain naturally "fermented" products such as apple cider vinegar and dinner wines consumed in moderation. Also, as Dr.

Blaylock explains in his book, truly natural fermentation by specific probiotic or "friendly" bacteria on certain whole food extracts also has proven to be extremely beneficial and helpful in protecting the human cell from the potential ravages of chemically altered excess free glutamate excito-toxins.   (A very fine example of this is a product named Core Food provided by exclusive formulation by a company called Sageant LLC, Bozeman, Montana.)

It is only when certain genetically modified bacteria is used in the fermentation process that potentially deadly excessive amounts of excitatory amino acids are produced.   The abnormal folding of chemically altered amino acid chains in protein molecules may also be the primary mechanism in the mutation of proteins into deadly prions, which is the basic sequence of events in the mad-cow phenomenon and the human version, variant CJD syndrome – which is currently incurable and 100% lethal.

Keep in mind that Ajinomoto and its sister Japanese Corporate giant Monsanto Inc. have been formulating and selling livestock feed additives for decades in America, Canada, the U.K. and Europe. Closely related to MSG, these additives are similarly chemically altered amino acids that have been engineered to fatten up livestock quickly and efficiently at the feedlot, just prior to slaughter. Ask any rancher. What makes him more profit, a skinny, wiry range steer, or a rotund, obese, artificially fattened heifer with marbled, fat meat?

Could such altered amino acids possibly be a causative factor in the Bovine Spongiform mutations observed in the brains of Mad-Cows? Since BSE (mad-cow disease) made its appearance in the same decade following the introductions of such bio-engineered feed additives, would this at least merit a single international, objective research study? **An open-minded objective person would no doubt agree.**

So, are you a victim of MSG toxicity or not? Do you know for a fact if you or your family members are actually overweight or obese? The clinical definition of obesity is "an excessively high amount of body fat or adipose tissue in relation to lean body mass."[i] The actual amount of body fat (or adiposity) is concerned with both the distribution of fat throughout the body as well as the actual size of the adipose (fatty) tissue deposits. The distribution of body fat can be estimated by a number of techniques including skinfold measures, waist-to-hip circumference ratios, or techniques such as ultrasound, computed tomography, or MRI (magnetic resonance imaging). The national standard for determining obesity, however, is the calculation of your Body Mass Index, or BMI.

Individuals with a BMI of 25 to 29.9 are considered to be overweight, while individuals with a BMI of 30 or more are considered to be obese. This is a vital statistic for you to consider, because obese individuals with a BMI of 30 or more are at much higher risk for many diseases, including diabetes, heart disease, high blood pressure, and cancers.

It is a very good idea to know you and your loved one's BMI and monitor it often. To calculate your BMI, divide your weight by your height in inches times your height in inches, then multiply the result by 703. For instance if you are 5 feet in height (12X5=60 inches) and you weigh 160 pounds, your BMI is calculated by dividing 160 (your weight) by 3600 (60 inches times 60 inches). This number

(.0444444) is then multiplied by 703 and the BMI index is thus calculated at 31.24, an obese number.   If your BMI is over 25, chances are excellent that you have been victimized by MSG toxicity, just as the helpless mice and rats in lab cages worldwide are made unnaturally obese just by eating normal portions.   The bottom line folks, is obesity in America may not be entirely due to over-eating.   It may not be your "fault" AT ALL!

---

[1] Centers for Disease Control, NRC p114; Stunkard p14)

Chapter 3

The Trial

Few people are capable of expressing with equanimity opinions which differ from the prejudices of their social environment. Most people are even incapable of forming such opinions.
- Albert Einstein

The large multinational conglomerate, Ajinomoto Inc. which produces much of the world's supply of altered amino acid exitotoxins named MSG and its peptide cousin Aspartame, would like you to believe their propaganda that these products are benign, harmless, completely natural, and 100% safe. Of course, they would demand such unquestioning loyalty – because they literally have a Trillion-Yen (100 Billion US Dollar) annual net income stream to protect.[i] But a careful study and review of Drs. Schwartz and Blaylock's work clearly indicates otherwise.

Isn't it interesting that on Ajinomoto's website, they proudly announce that they soon will be introducing a patented DRUG (another chemically altered amino acid) that will artificially regulate insulin levels in diabetics. The pharmaceutical industry is projecting that within a decade; this new wonder drug may eliminate the need for insulin injections by diabetics. HMMMM – let's see. There appears to be a pattern emerging here. It's called Problem, Reaction, and Solution. A group of individuals create a Problem, (in this case, an increased risk for Diabetes), then they monitor and even contribute to the prescribed Reaction in the mainstream press and media, and then of course miraculously come up with the Solution (a wonder-drug that does not HEAL diabetes mellitus, only fools the body once again into thinking that insulin levels are normal!) Undoubtedly, both the drug product that is a causative factor in the problem, as well as the wonder-drug solution both are designed to generate massive profits. No wonder Ajinomoto's net income increases 9% every year after being adjusted for inflation.[ii]

The marketing agents of Ajinomoto's MSG here in America will quickly point out and argue that MSG has been used for over 50 years in Japan. If it is so dangerous, then why are the Japanese people so very healthy? In order to answer that argument, I submit that we need to define the term "healthy". While it is true that the Japanese have a 3-year longer life expectancy than their American counterparts, I would definitely not declare that they are "healthier". In fact, some deeper research absolutely strengthens the links between MSG, Aspartame, and chronic obesity, diabetes, and other deadly diseases.

In Ajinomoto's 2004 corporate report, they state that the countries that have consumed the most MSG (i.e. generated the most profit) are Japan, the United States, and Germany respectively. [iii] In fact, Ajinomoto has formed wholly owned corporate subsidiaries, Ajinomoto USA, and Ajinomoto Deutschland that oversee the production and marketing of MSG in America and Europe. Last year, these three countries substantially increased their profit margins for their mother company. Specifically, sales increased 4.3% in Japan, 10.5% in Germany, and 11.5% in the U.S.[iv] If more people were consuming increasing quantities of MSG in these countries over the last 30 years, would it not make sense that specific disease rates such as obesity, diabetes, and certain cancers would increase in the same countries as well if MSG was a causative factor?

According to the International Diabetes Federation statistics, this is exactly the case.   In 2003, the five countries with the largest numbers of persons with diabetes were India (35.5 million), China (23.8 million) the United States (16 million) Russia (9.7 million) and Japan (6.7 million).[v] When adjusted to a per capita basis, Japan is number 1, the United States is second, and Germany is third.   So, let's see, the three nations that are the largest consumers of MSG on planet earth, also have the most obese diabetics as well. Unfortunately, there are even more smoking guns to be concerned about.

According to statistics compiled by the World Health Organization in 2003, Japan, America, and Germany lead the way in many other disease categories as well.   Japan led the way with mortalities caused by cerebral infarction, followed by the United States and Germany.[vi]   Also, Japan, the United States, and Germany led all developed countries in deaths caused by cancer of the liver, gallbladder, gum and mouth, other and "unspecified parts of the biliary tract".   These three countries also led the world in deaths caused by cancer of the stomach, ureter, rectum, and renal pelvis, as well as cancer of the thymus, which of course is the thermostat of health and vitality of the entire immune system![vii]   If one didn't know better, one could easily be led to assume by these statistics that the people living in these three countries are being systematically poisoned to death. But there is still more.

Japan, the United States and Germany lead all developed countries in deaths from interstitial pulmonary heart diseases, strokes, and Parkinson's Disease. In all, these three countries lead the way in over 60 different disease mortality categories, often in both actual numbers of deaths as well as per capita statistics. Perhaps most telling is the fact that Japan still leads the world in suicide deaths by middle-aged individuals.[viii] Could it be that Kamikaze is still fashionable in Japan, especially when MSG induced mental depression with feelings of hopeless failure are added to the mix?

Isn't it just a remarkable set of coincidences that every health issue raised by Dr. Blaylock in his book *Excitotoxins* is borne out by the international statistics? But the biggest question is, why is the FDA allowing these large multinational conglomerates to continue to market such clearly dangerous products? Why is this scandal not being addressed in the halls of Congress, and the United Nations? Could it be that Big Business Buries the Truth?

A recent publication entitled *Diabetes and Obesity: Time to Act*, authored by the International Diabetes Federation (IDF) and the International Association for the Study of Obesity (IASO) sums it all up very succinctly: "The twin epidemics of diabetes and obesity are rising dramatically around the world and urgent action is needed if a global public health crisis is to be avoided."

Again, what is meant by "urgent action"? I submit that this means outlawing the food additives that are linked to Obesity and Diabetes – specifically Aspartame and MSG. Humans are NOT feedlot cattle or swine to be chemically fattened up before the slaughter. Or are we?

Of course, Ajinomoto is not the only corporate entity to employ such questionable practices. Consider the case of pharmaceutical giant American Home Products.

During the early 90's, American Home Products (AHP Inc.) found a brilliant way to capitalize on the obesity problem faced by Americans, and others worldwide. They found that after creating obese mice and rats in their laboratory (by injecting them with MSG, remember?), they could introduce a couple of Central Nervous System (CNS) stimulant chemical drugs that would automatically raise the metabolic factors of the test animals so that they would systematically lose the MSG induced weight gains. The protocol was amazingly effective, and an incredibly easy sell because this "miracle weight loss" happened without having to exercise. The chemicals magically reduced fat cells.

But, unfortunately, there was one major drawback. There usually are side effects when you fool around with Mother Nature. A certain percentage of the test rodents developed PERMANENT damage to their hearts. This held true in repeated tests. AHP Inc. had a dilemma. Could they afford the risk involved with introducing this miracle weight loss prescription formula to the general public, knowing full well that it would cause a certain percentage of the people to experience permanently disabling heart damage?

AHP Executives were (and are) not stupid. They knew very well the Billions of Dollars they could quickly generate by the sensationalism of such a weight loss drug. So they did what all good business executives are trained to do at Ivy League business schools. They BUDGETED FOR THE ESTIMATED LOSS. In other words, in their corporate boardroom, they actually projected the billions they would make, then set aside a portion of their projections for a settlement of claims for the inevitable heart damage claims that they would receive. This, you see, was only shrewd business planning. I am confident that they factored in a larger purchase price to reflect the liability they knew full well they were creating. Of course, they employed a number of competent attorneys in their "legal department" as well. With any amount of luck, they could defer any liability. This is yet another example of Big Business Burying the Truth.

Sure enough, the Fen-Phen craze hit America in a very big way. Strategically placed advertisements in most newspapers and magazines, as well as radio and TV paid off in a very handsome fashion. Within a few short months, AHP Inc. was making hundreds of millions dollars more net profits, and their stock soared. All was well, the AHP top executives were happy, the politicians in D.C. were happy because tax revenues increased, Media Executives were happy because of the massive advertising dollars spent, the doctors were happy because plump housewives and their couch potato husbands had to pay for an office visit to get the Fen-Phen prescription, and the AHP stockholders were even happier. Everyone was happy.

Everyone, that is, except America's attorneys. AHP Inc. execs did not calculate correctly how much it was going to take to make America's attorneys happy. The claims of heart damage began pouring in, and more than a few heart surgeons refused to remain quiet about the cause of the damage in their patients. Fen-Phen was immediately targeted as a potential cause of the problems, but initially there was no real "smoking gun".

Soon, however, the proverbial defecating fecal matter impacted with force on the oscillating blade. There was an internal leak at AHP Inc. Word of the earlier studies got out. It was eventually proven in a court of law that AHP knew that the drug was problematic – and yet marketed it anyway. The floodgates were opened, and a torrent of claims flooded AHP Inc.'s legal department. In a massive class action settlement that as of the summer of 2004 is still not completely settled, hundreds of enterprising attorneys have made millions in assisting their clients to receive compensation. Yet, the sad fact remains that Fen-Phen still appears to have made AHP a lot of money, in spite of the terrible publicity and widespread heartache their product created.

I would like to submit to the AHP executives that no amount of compensation should replace a human heart. How tragic that you apparently placed corporate profits ahead of the health concerns of the public. You, a very Big Business, Buried the Truth! Especially when you were apprised of the risks and apparently knew full well that it WOULD cause heart problems. You just did not know for sure exactly HOW MANY hearts would be damaged.

But there are still a lot of unanswered questions. How did AHP Inc.'s Fen-Phen get FDA approval in the first place? Did they not analyze the test reports? Were the reports the FDA received from AHP genuinely accurate or were they fabricated?

It would seem to this American citizen that there should be at least some shouldering of blame and liability by the FDA. You know something? If I buy a big, tough watchdog to guard my property, and while looking mean and growling once in a while, he goes to sleep every time the thieves are at work – whom do I blame? Do I become upset at the dog itself, or the trainer who sold it to me? The American Public is looking to the FDA to screen drugs such as Fen-Phen – where did things go wrong there? Can we really trust the FDA, or in the real world are their services for sale for the highest pharmaceutical bidder?? Does the FDA subscribe to the maxim that Big Business Buries the Truth?

In the case of MSG's 1st cousin Aspartame, which is a manufactured peptide, it appears that FDA approval for Nutrasweet was procured in much the same manner. Nutrasweet, the American name for Aspartame, was under contract to be produced and marketed in America by a company by the name of G.D. Searle. In 1975, G.D. Searle applied with the FDA to have Aspartame approved as a sugar alternative. But their application hit a big snag. FDA Commissioner Dr. Alexander Schmidt actually appointed a special task force to investigate Searle and their testing procedures on Aspartame. Apparently, G.D. Searle had failed to report studies that showed that Aspartame caused tumors and epileptic seizures in test monkeys and lab mice.

In 1977, the FDA task force did indeed find and subsequently report that G.D. Searle had been fraudulent in their reported research on the safety of Aspartame. In fact, records show that the FDA's chief legal counsel, Richard Merrill, even went so far as to formally request that U.S. Attorney Samuel Skinner convene a Grand Jury to further investigate and possibly indict G.D. Searle executives on criminal charges. As happens all too often in big business, especially in big government, neither Mr. Skinner nor his successor ever did convene that Grand Jury. By a mere quirk of purely coincidental fate however, both U.S. Attorneys ended up leaving their government positions in favor of fat salary increases from new positions with G.D. Searle's law firm. Big Business once again successfully Buried the Truth.

In 1980, another courageously honest physician named Dr. John Olney had examined the dangers of "excitotoxins" such as MSG and Aspartame. He successfully managed to bring together a Public Board of Inquiry to examine the dangers and toxicity levels of Aspartame. In the same year, the Board unanimously voted to demand the FDA reject Aspartame until more extensive testing could be performed concerning the apparent links to Aspartame and brain tumor growths and Alzheimer's Disease. The FDA had little choice. They concurred with the Board of Inquiry's findings.

For a few weeks, it looked as if it was a sure bet that the American public would be protected from the toxic ravages of Aspartame. But G.D. Searle was not licked yet. They had a very aggressive board of directors, and a passel of impatient stockholders to protect. At the height of the Aspartame controversy in 1977, Searle hired themselves a new Chief Executive Officer. His resume was most impressive. He had extensive government contacts, as he worked as a trusted, high-level presidential staff member under both the Nixon and Ford administrations. Funny how this new CEO kept his job with Gerald Ford when he was constantly on the hot seat for his insider knowledge of the Watergate scandal – his services were obviously extremely valuable on Capitol Hill. His name: Donald Rumsfeld.

Mr. Rumsfeld you see, had obvious business savvy and was extremely "well connected" – that was why G.D. Searle recruited him. He had seen the profit projections that a sweetener with zero calories would generate. I am confident that he also knew how valuable a brain-deadening agent could be in a corrupt government's hands. In short, he was (and still is) very skilled in the art of Burying the Truth.

In January of 1981, a Hollywood actor named Ronald Reagan brought a new brand of entrepreneurial spirit into the oval office. Within a very short time, it became clear that Mr. Reagan was more interested in protecting favored stockholders and lobbyists than the general public. After all as Mr. Reagan so eloquently and forcefully declared, improve Wall Street profits, and you increase tax revenues as well – and "trickle-down Reaganomics" was born.

Within a very short time, Searle CEO Rumsfeld gained a private audience with the new president. Immediately thereafter, CEO Rumsfeld put in a new application to the FDA requesting that they declare Aspartame safe as a food additive, instead of a stand-alone sugar substitute drug. In March of 1981, FDA Commissioner Jere Goyan refused to totally buckle in to the political pressures of the new administration, and instead of giving Aspartame the rubber stamp of approval, he established a special 5-member panel of independent scientists to objectively review the issues outlined and delineated in the 1980 Board of Inquiry. This was the obviously honest and correct move. Unfortunately, the 5-member panel would never complete their review. The following month, in April, an enraged Reagan replaced Jere Goyan with Arthur Hull Hayes, Jr. as FDA Commissioner. Two months later, Commissioner Hayes somehow ignored all previous Board of Inquiry findings and publicly declared that Aspartame (G.D. Searle's Nutrasweet) could be safely added to food and drink. Exactly one year later, without any further study, the FDA made it totally and completely legal to add this mutated peptide drug to soft drinks and other diet, "low-fat" products. Of course, as a direct result, G.D. Searle stock soared, and CEO Rumsfeld received a hefty Christmas bonus – as well as an unprecedented golden parachute package for a job well done. Big Business Buried the Truth. Is this not criminal?

Too bad that President Reagan was more concerned about corporate profits than his own health. Between the aspartame in certain little "low-fat" candies that he became fond of and consumed by the hundreds, as well as the diet soft drinks he preferred to consumed, little wonder he had a hard time remembering what happened with Ollie North and the Iran/Contra arms for hostages scandal that elevated him into the presidency. One can only wonder how much his love of aspartame led to the onset of his Alzheimer's Disease. One can also only wonder how involved Rumsfeld was in brokering the arms deals with the contras, as the South and Central America countries were one of his "areas of expertise" under the Ford Administration 4 years earlier.

The rest of the story of Aspartame is literally history now. Aspartame, aka Nutrasweet has literally made its mark on the entire world, and absolutely guaranteed the financial success of Donald Rumsfeld's company, as well as Ajinomoto Inc. in Japan. Mr.

Rumsfeld must have really been impressive to President Reagan, for just a few years later, he was appointed special envoy to the Middle East in 1983. Two years later, in 1985, Rumsfeld returned to G.D. Searle just long enough to oversee the sale of G.D. Searle to Monsanto Corp. Once again, CEO Rumsfeld received a multi-million dollar bonus and benefit package.

With chemical giant Monsanto in control of Nutrasweet, sales dramatically escalated. By the time George H.W. Bush took over the White House, Diet Sodas were suddenly extremely popular. "Just one Calorie" ads and jingles were seen and heard every hour on TV and Radio. And who were the target consumers? Young people who wanted to maintain their trim, youthful appearances. The same young people who George Bush Sr. called on to help liberate Kuwait from the Evil Emperor/Ruthless Dictator Saddam Hussein in Operation Desert Storm. The same young people who now are suffering disabilities referred to as Gulf War Syndrome or GWS.

The Veterans Administration reports that there are hundreds of thousands of Gulf War Veterans and their immediate family members who are reporting symptoms remarkably similar to Chronic Fatigue Syndrome and Fibromyalgia. Specifically, "a set of nonspecific complaints with emphasis on Central Nervous System (CNS) impairment." This includes extremely painful muscles, severe headaches, dizziness, weakness, fainting, and sexual dysfunctions. To this day, nobody in the medical community is willing to publicly declare the root cause of GWS. Surely, our US Military has some very good ideas?? Some "experts" say that those sneaky Iraqis perhaps subjected the troops to some sort of covert chemical weapon attack. I believe the "experts" are half right. I believe those who suffer from Gulf War Syndrome are indeed the victims of a covert chemical weapon attack, but it did not come from the Iraqis.

During Operation Desert Storm, the coalition forces were promised the very best in logistic support. And for the most part, they got it. The mess tents were supplied with the very best foods America had to offer – fresh meats and vegetables along with crates of chips and snack foods were plentiful – and so was soda pop, especially diet drinks – in aluminum cans. Since the refrigeration units were primarily used to store the perishable meats and vegetables, untold numbers of pallet loads of diet soda drinks laced with the drug Aspartame were left to swelter in the hot Persian Gulf desert sun for days, weeks, and months before they were consumed. Here is how our service men and women came under covert chemical attack by another "Secret Assassin" a ninja of taste.

Aspartame, as a mutated peptide, does not remain stable for long. At 86 degrees Fahrenheit (well below the normal human body temperature of 98.6) Aspartame has been shown to transform into a very hazardous chemical called formaldehyde. Formaldehyde when consumed accumulates in the human liver and has been linked to every symptom consistent with Chronic Fatigue Syndrome and Fibromyalgia, as well as cancerous tumors and such lethal conditions as Non-Hodgkin's Lymphoma. At temperatures above 100 degrees, the amounts of methanol and formaldehyde formed are even greater.

It doesn't take much imagination to picture what would happen to the formaldehyde content of semi-loads of diet sodas with Aspartame baking in the 120+ degree Kuwaiti sun, where extremely thirsty soldiers could drink dozens of them every day. Would it be too extreme to declare that these soldiers could easily experience long-term negative effects from such chemical contamination? Moreover, how many milligrams of MSG were injected into our soldiers veins with the myriad of vaccinations they required before going overseas??

Isn't it also an extremely ironic coincidence that the same corporate CEO-turned-cabinet-staffer who was largely responsible for placing the chemical Aspartame in those simmering diet drinks, is now the very same Secretary of Defense who is once again asking the nation's armed forces to be placed in harm's way in Iraq? One can only wonder how many more diet sodas are broiling in the Iraqi sun in some supply depot in Iraq as this book is written.

In 1985, prior to the 1st Persian Gulf War, Senator Howard Metzenbaum conducted an investigation of Searle and Nutrasweet. He independently verified the truths outlined in the pages of this book, and felt so strongly about the problem that he drafted a bill. Unfortunately, it never made it out of the Senate Labor and Human Resources Committee, for reasons that should be fairly obvious. Big business buries the truth, and the pharmaceutical lobbyists wielded their incredible power. If only Metzenbaum's bill had become law, countless lives and illnesses could undoubtedly have been spared. See the addendum for the verbatim copy of the bill, and correspondence between Senator Orrin Hatch, Labor and Human Resources Committee Chariman, and Metzenbaum in 1986.

The reason why I am explaining the details about Aspartame is the fact that Aspartame's chemical structure often causes many of the same toxic symptoms as MSG. Specifically, Aspartame often affects the same neurons in the body that MSG does. In the digestive tract, Aspartame has been shown to break down into an amino acid called phenylalanine. There is a certain percentage of the population that has an inherited condition called phenylketonuria, which is a big long word that simply means their bodies cannot metabolize certain amino acids – and so Aspartame becomes highly toxic to these individuals. Pregnant mothers with this condition who ingest Aspartame during their pregnancy have been shown to have a 93% chance that their baby will be born mentally retarded, and a 72% chance that their child will be born with a significantly smaller brain. Where are the FDA warning labels on drinks with Aspartame? Where are the nutritionists explaining the links to MSG and obesity? Why are the studies and reports continuing to be hidden? Why does Ajinomoto produce both products, MSG and Aspartame, without liability? Big Business Buries the Truth.

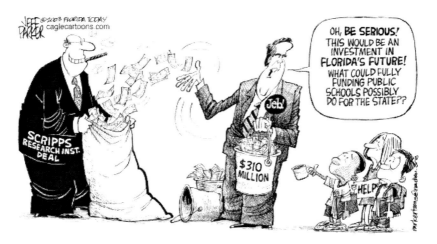

ASPARTAME, THE SILENT KILLER, ANOTHER "SECRET ASSASSIN"
2 "Must-Read" Reports

Report One: (written in 1999 by a colleague of Dr. Roberts)

Alzheimers is not only triggered by aluminum although it is one reason for the disease. Dr. H.J. Roberts has done 30 years of research on Alzheimers and has just published a book on it called DEFENSE AGAINST ALZHEIMERS DISEASE (for the book call 1-800-814-9800). It has been nominated for a Pulitzer and is a very knowledgeable and incredible book written with great dignity, understanding and compassion. Dr. Roberts was in Atlanta giving a seminar and went into some things that can trigger Alzheimers. When aspartame, (marketed as NutraSweet, Equal, Spoonful, etc.) was approved, Dr. Roberts noticed a big difference in his diabetic and multiple sclerosis patients. (Dr. Roberts is a diabetic specialist.) They showed memory loss, confusion, and serious vision problems. He goes into this in his book. Alzheimers is a 20th century disease and is now the fourth leading cause of death in adults in the U.S. (4 million victims.)

Dr. Roberts says that the two amino acids in aspartame are neurotoxic without the other amino acids in protein (phenylalanine and aspartic acid). They go past the blood brain barrier and deteriorate the neurons of the brain. This is the cause of Alzheimers. Dr. Roberts says, in his opinion, that NutraSweet is escalating Alzheimers. There are 250,000 new cases each year and 100,000 deaths. Fifty percent of all patients in nursing homes are Alzheimers patients (including mature baby boomers). A couple of days ago a nursing assistant told me she was just shocked that now 30 year old women are being admitted with Alzheimers.

Aspartame is nothing but a chemical poison. It has methyl ester in it that becomes methanol (wood alcohol), and in the body (at 86 degrees F) it converts to formaldehyde and formic acid (ant sting poison) and causes metabolic acidosis. (Merck Index, pg 143)

Aspartame is absolutely disastrous for a diabetic patient even though it is recommended by the American Diabetic Association, but that's only because the ADA is funded by Monsanto, the chemical manufacturer of Aspartame. Dr. Roberts has been a member for almost forty years and gave them an abstract of diabetic aspartame reactors, but they refused to publish it. It was however published in the periodical Clinical Research (Vol. 36, No. 3, 1988, 489A). I suspect the ADA can't warn the diabetics this is a poison and at the same time, continue to take big money from its manufacturer, Monsanto. You can be sure however, that on or around October 1 every year, the NutraSweet Company (Monsanto) will continue to sponsor walk-a-thons for the ADA and distribute Equal trademark logo shirts.

One big problem diabetics face is diabetic retinopathy – i.e. the deterioration of their eyesight. Many physicians do not realize that when diabetics are consuming aspartame, what is really happening is that the patients are going blind. The very same methanol (wood alcohol) that blinded and killed so many skid row drunks during the prohibition era, converts to formaldehyde in the retina of the eye. That's why so many diabetics bleed and have retinal detachments. It's so very tragic, and is also so very preventable in many cases.

Dr. Russell Blaylock, neurosurgeon, wrote a book titled: EXCITOTOXINS: THE TASTE THAT KILLS. His research as published in the book says that the ingredients in NutraSweet (aspartame) literally stimulate the neurons of the brain to death, causing brain damage in varying degrees. This is even written on the back cover of the book! He also declares that aspartame can trigger diabetes. It is really no wonder that there are so very many diabetics in this country, and more being diagnosed every day!

In August, 1995, the FDA listed the following symptoms from the consumption of aspartame: Headaches, dizziness or balance problems, change in mood quality or level, vomiting and nausea, abdominal pain and cramps, change in vision, diarrhea, seizures and convulsions, change in heart rate, itching, change in sensation (numbness, tingling), grand mal seizures, local swelling, change in activity level, difficulty in breathing, oral sensory changes, change in menstrual pattern, other localized pain and tenderness, other urogenital problems, body temperature changes, swallowing difficulty, other metabolic problems, joint and bone pain, speech impairment, miscellaneous gastrointestinal problems, chest pain, other musculo-skeletal problems, fainting, sore throat, other cardiovascular problems, change in taste, difficulty with urination, other respiratory problems, edema, change in hearing, change in perspiration patterns, eye irritation, unspecified muscle tremors, petit mal, change in body weight, change in thirst or water intake, unconsciousness and coma, wheezing, constipation, other extremity pain, problems with bleeding, unsteady gait, coughing, blood glucose disorders, blood pressure changes, changes in skin and nail coloration, change in hair or nails, excessive phlegm production, sinus problems, simple partial seizures, hallucinations, dysmenorrehea, dental problems, change in smell, **DEATH,** other blood and lymphatic problems, eczema, complex partial seizures, swollen lymph nodes, hematuria, shortness of breath, difficulties with pregnancy, developmental retardation in children, change in breast size or tenderness, change in sexual function, shock, conjunctivitis, dilating eyes.

QUESTION: If you saw these many adverse reactions listed in the Physician's Desk Reference (PDR) of drugs, WOULD YOU SERIOUSLY HAVE TO RECONSIDER TAKING IT, EVEN THOUGH PRESCRIBED BY YOUR FAMILY DOCTOR??

Attention folks, in actuality, Aspartame IS IN FACT A DRUG!! It was discovered by a Seattle chemist who was testing different chemicals, to try and find relief for peptic ulcers.

Notice also, how the FDA just happened to throw the word DEATH in the middle of all of those other side-effect 'symptoms'. What a nice little alternative to white, refined sugar. Barbara Mullarkey, a journalist in Oak Park, Illinois, has also written about aspartame since it was approved – and has also written about the symptoms the drug induces. In other words, the FDA's list is quite accurate. One article she wrote played on this, and was titled: DEATH: THE ULTIMATE 'SYMPTOM'!

Keep in mind when congressional hearings were held in Washington on this subject, aspartame was only in a few hundred products. Today, the patent has expired and it is in over 5,000 products – and growing daily. Today you have this wonderful 'drug' in your coffee, in your soda, ice cream, jello gelatin, gum, over the counter medications as well as prescription drugs, and it is now even in baked goods. You absolutely cannot heat aspartame safely, because when you do it becomes a veritable witches brew of 'breakdown products', but the FDA forgot to mention this when they approved it's use in baked goods back in 1993!!

Is there any reasonable doubt why aspartame is triggering so many neurological symptoms and disease? Anything that changes the brain chemistry is potentially disastrous! It really does a number also on Parkinson's patients, primarily because it changes the dopamine level.

Whoever said that the FDA is not trustworthy is absolutely correct. This in my opinion is one of the greatest atrocities a branch of the federal government has ever committed in the history of this country. Initially, there was so much legitimate opposition to the approval of this drug, that the FDA set up a Board of Inquiry. The board studied the issue, and gave a recommendation not to approve aspartame because it was shown to cause brain tumors and grand mal seizures in lab animals (just for starters). However, Dr. Arthur Hull Hayes, head of the FDA, quietly overruled his own Board of Inquiry ------- and the drug was approved. Then conveniently and of course, just coincidentally, was hired and went to work for Searle's public relations firm and refused to talk to the press for over ten years. Monsanto of course, bought Searle in 1985, and Searle Pharmaceutical is the original patent holder (US patent 3492131)!

I firmly believe that aspartame is a major causative factor in the current widespread epidemic of chronic fatigue syndrome, systemic lupus, and fibromyalgia. Among other symptoms, methanol (the by-product of aspartame) primarily attacks and greatly weakens the immune system. People are also constantly being diagnosed with multiple sclerosis, when in reality they have methanol toxicity from their use of aspartame, which of course mimics the symptoms of MS! Many alert alternative practitioners report that if they get to them in time, many MS 'patients' have their symptoms reversed just by removing aspartame from their diets. If any one you know of consistently uses aspartame, and suffers from vision problems, headaches, slurring of words, numbness, cramps, shooting pains in the legs, vertigo, dizziness, tinnitus in the ears, joint pain, insomnia, etc. – they very likely are suffering from methanol toxicity. Be assured, methanol toxicity does in fact kill eventually!

Richard Wilson wrote the following in an Atlanta newspaper back in April, 1998: "Aspartame killed my wife. No words can express the agony and horror sweet Joyce endured. The poison destroyed her brain, ravaged her organs, and blinded her. She died at age 46 in 1996. ---------------- The makers of this poison considered her death an "acceptable cost of business". I'm a man without a wife because the NutraSweet Company is a business without a conscience."

Joyce Wilson had all of the symptoms of MS, was diagnosed as having it, when actually it was methanol toxicity from drinking too many diet drinks. When she died however, she was just like an Alzheimers victim with no memory. Up to that point, she tried her best to warn the world, and even testified before Congress. But of course, the deep pockets of Monsanto prevailed and her desperate pleas fell on deaf ears. Even the late Dr. Adrian Goss, FDA toxicologist, testified before Congress that aspartame violated the Delaney Amendment because "beyond a shadow of a doubt it caused cancer in lab animals." His last, dying words will never be forgotten: ***"If the FDA violates its own laws, who is left to protect the people?"*** The sad truth is, we really have no benevolent 'PROTECTOR', so we must warn each other.

Patricia Crane is yet another victim of NutraSweet. Her death was reported on CBN. It was mentioned that her autopsy (following a medically documented death like that of Joyce Wilson) was identical to that of Christina Onassis, a confirmed Diet Coke addict!! It's just not worth the risk folks. Millions of Americans are living a nightmare, and more often than not, their physicians don't recognize the symptoms because they don't associate them with aspartame/methanol poisoning. They have been brainwashed into accepting that aspartame is safe because the organizations (AMA, FDA, ADA, etc.) that have sold out to Monsanto have declared it to be so.

It is high time to look deeper, and declare the truth. I for one am dedicated to the belief that our society should not be satisfied until death, suffering, and wrongful disability are no longer considered "an acceptable cost of business". How long are we going to remain silent while major beverage companies are handsomely paying our colleges and universities to be the "official drink" on their campuses – 'official drinks' that are often laced with a potentially devastating 'drug'? Yet in the same breath, we vocalize and publicize victories in the ongoing 'war' against other drugs such as cocaine, heroin, marijuana, and methamphetamines. Is this not a shameful 'double standard' and absolute hypocrisy?

Report Two
(by a Medical Doctor)

"I have spent several days lecturing at the WORLD ENVIRONMENT CONFERENCE. The topic of my lecture was on "ASPARTAME marketed as 'NutraSweet', 'Equal', and 'Spoonful'." In the keynote address by the EPA, they announced that there was an epidemic of multiple sclerosis and systemic lupus, and they did not understand what toxin was causing this to be rampant across the United States. I explained that I was there to lecture on exactly that subject.

When the temperature of Aspartame exceeds 86 degrees F, the wood alcohol in Aspartame converts to formaldehyde and then to formic acid, which in turn causes metabolic acidosis. (Formic acid is the poison found in the sting of fire ants.) The methanol toxicity mimics multiple sclerosis; thus people were being diagnosed with having multiple sclerosis in error.

Multiple Sclerosis is not a death sentence, however methanol toxicity is. In the case of systemic lupus, we are finding it has become almost as rampant as multiple sclerosis, especially among Diet Coke and Diet Pepsi drinkers. Also, with methanol toxicity, the victims usually drink three to four 12 oz. cans of them per day, some even more. In the cases of systemic lupus, which is triggered by Aspartame, the victim usually does not know that the Aspartame is the culprit. The victim continues its use, aggravating the lupus to such a degree that sometimes it becomes life threatening. When we get people off the Aspartame, those with systemic lupus usually become asymptomatic. Unfortunately, we cannot currently reverse this disease.

On the other hand, in the case of those diagnosed with Multiple Sclerosis, (when in reality, the disease is methanol toxicity), most of the symptoms disappear. We have seen cases where their vision has returned and even their hearing has returned. This also applies to cases of tinnitus. During a lecture I said, "If you are using Aspartame (NutraSweet, Equal, Spoonful, etc.) and you suffer from fibromyalgia symptoms, spasms, shooting pains, numbness in your legs, cramps, vertigo, dizziness, headaches, tinnitus, joint pains, depression, anxiety attacks, slurred speech, blurred vision, or memory loss – you probably have Aspartame Disease!"

People were jumping up during the lecture saying, "I've got this, it is reversible?" It is absolutely rampant. Some of the speakers at my lecture even were suffering from these symptoms. In a lecture attended by the Ambassador of Uganda, he told us that their sugar industry is adding Aspartame! He continued by saying that one of the industry's leader's sons could no longer walk – due in part by product usage!

We have a serious problem facing us. Even a stranger came up to Dr. Espisto (one of my speakers) and myself and said, 'Could you tell me why so many people seem to be coming down with MS?' During a visit to a hospice, a nurse said that six of her friends, who were heavy Diet Coke addicts, had all been diagnosed with MS. This is beyond coincidence.

Here is the problem. There were Congressional Hearings when Aspartame was included in only 100 different products. Since this initial hearing, there have been two subsequent hearings, but to no avail. Nothing has been done. The drug and chemical lobbies have very deep pockets. Now there are over 5,000 products containing this chemical, and the PATENT HAS EXPIRED!!!!

Aspartame can now be found in:
- Instant breakfasts, gelatin desserts, soft drinks and pop
- Breath mints, juice beverages, tabletop sweeteners
- Cereals, laxatives, tea beverages.
- Sugar-free chewing gum, multivitamins, instant coffees and teas
- Cocoa mixes, milk drinks, topping mixes
- Coffee beverages, pharmaceuticals and health supplements
- Wine coolers, frozen desserts, shake mixes and yogurts

At the time of this first hearing, people were going blind. The methanol in the Aspartame converts to formaldehyde in the retina of the eye. Formaldehyde is grouped in the same class of drugs as CYANIDE and ARSENIC – DEADLY POISONS!! Unfortunately, it just takes longer to quietly kill, but it is killing people and causing all kinds of neurological problems nevertheless. Aspartame changes the brain's chemistry. It is the reason for severe seizures. This drug changes the dopamine level in the brain. Imagine what this drug does to patients suffering from Parkinson's Disease. This drug also causes birth defects.

There is absolutely no reason to take this product. It is NOT A DIET PRODUCT!!!! The Congressional record said, "It makes you crave carbohydrates and [they] will make you fat." Dr. Roberts stated that when he got patients off Aspartame, their average weight loss was 19 pounds per person. The formaldehyde stores in the fat cells, particularly in the hips and thighs.

Aspartame is especially deadly for diabetics. All physicians know what wood alcohol will do to a diabetic. We find that physicians believe that they have patients with retinopathy, when in fact their blindness is caused by the Aspartame. The Aspartame keeps the blood sugar level out of control, causing many patients to go into coma. Unfortunately, many have died.

People were telling us at the Conference of the American College of Physicians that they had relatives that switched from saccharin to an Aspartame product and how that relative had eventually gone into a coma. Their physicians could not get the blood sugar levels under control. Thus the patients suffered acute memory loss and eventually coma and death.

Memory loss is due to the fact that aspartic acid and phenylalanine are neurotoxic without the other amino acids found in protein. Thus it goes past the blood brain barrier and deteriorates the neurons of the brain.

Dr. H.L. Roberts, diabetic specialist and world expert on aspartame poisoning, has also written a book entitled "DEFENSE AGAINST ALZHEIMER'S DISEASE". Dr. Roberts tells how aspartame poisoning is escalating Alzheimers disease and indeed it is. As the hospice nurse told me, women are being admitted at 30 years of age with Alzheimer's Disease. Dr. Roberts and I will be writing a position paper with some case histories and will post it on the Internet. According to the Conference of the American College of Physicians, "We are talking about a plague of neurological diseases caused by this deadly poison."

Dr. Roberts realized what was happening when aspartame was first marketed. He said, "many diabetic patients presented memory loss, confusion, and severe vision loss." At the Conference of the American College of Physicians, doctors admitted that they did not know. They had wondered why seizures were rampant (the phenylalanine in aspartame breaks down the seizure threshold and depletes serotonin, which causes manic depression, panic attacks, rage and violence). Just before the conference, I received a fax from Norway, asking for a possible antidote for this poison because they are experiencing so many problems in their country.

This "poison" is now available in 90-plus countries worldwide. Fortunately, we had speakers and ambassadors at the Conference from different nations who have pledged their help. We ask that you help too.

Copy this article and warn everyone you know. Take anything that contains aspartame back to the store. Take the "NO ASPARTAME TEST" and send us your case history. I assure you that MONSANTO, the creator of aspartame, knows how deadly it is. They fund the American Diabetes Association, American Dietetic Association Congress, and the Conference of the American College of Physicians.

The New York Times, on November 15, 1996, ran an article on how the American Dietetic Association takes money from the food industry to endorse their products. Therefore, they cannot criticize any additives or tell about their link to MONSANTO. How bad is this?

We told a mother who had a child on NutraSweet to get off the product. The child was having grand mal seizures every day. The mother called her physician, who called the ADA, who told the doctor not to take the child off the NutraSweet. We are still trying to convince the mother that the aspartame is causing the seizures. Every time we get someone off aspartame, the seizures stop. If the baby dies, you know whose fault it is, and what we are up against. THERE ARE 92 DOCUMETED SYMPTOMS OF

ASPARTAME POISONING, RANGING FROM COMA TO DEATH!! The majority of them are all neurological, because the aspartame destroys the nervous system.

Aspartame disease is partially the cause to what is behind some of the mystery of the Desert Storm health problems. The burning tongue and other problems discussed in over 60 cases can be directly related to the consumption of an aspartame product. Several thousand pallets of diet drinks were shipped to the Desert Storm troops. (Remember heat can liberate the methanol from the aspartame at 86 degrees F.) These diet drinks sat in the 120 degree F. Arabian sun for weeks at a time on pallets. The service men and women drank them all day long. All of their symptoms are identical to aspartame poisoning.

Dr. Roberts says "consuming Aspartame at the time of conception can cause birth defects." The phenylalanine concentrates in the placenta, causing mental retardation, according to Dr. Louis Elsas, Pediatrician Professor – Genetics, at Emory University in his testimony before Congress. In the original lab tests, animals developed brain tumors (phenylalanine breaks down into DXP, a brain tumor agent). When Dr. Espisto was lecturing on aspartame, I, a physician in the audience and a neurosurgeon, said, "when they remove brain tumors, they have found high levels of aspartame in them!"

Stevia, a sweet FOOD, NOT AN ADDITIVE, which helps in the metabolism of sugar, which would be ideal for diabetics, has now been approved as a dietary supplement by the FDA. For years the FDA has outlawed this sweet food because of their loyalty to Monsanto.

If it says "SUGAR FREE" on the label – DO NOT EVEN THINK ABOUT CONSUMING IT!!!! Senator Howard Metzenbaum wrote a bill that would have warned all infants, pregnant mothers and children of the dangers of Aspartame. The bill would have also instilled independent studies on the problems existing in the population, (seizures, changes in brain chemistry, changes in neurological and behavioral symptoms. Sadly, the bill was killed by the powerful drug and chemical lobbies, letting loose the hounds of disease and death on an unsuspecting public. Since the Conference of the American College of Physicians, we hope to have the help of some world leaders in this battle. Again, please help us too. There are millions of people out there who must be warned. Please let them know about this very vital information."
Dr. R. B.

The TRUTH is that between the years 1965 and 1982 over 4 MILLION new, distinct, inorganic chemical compounds such as aspartame and propylene glycol were created and over 250,000 new formulations have been created each year since then. Approximately 3,000 of these new compounds have been added to our processed foods, and over 700 have been found in municipal drinking water supplies. 400 of these brand new compounds have even been found in human tissue. Even though it is becoming increasingly difficult to find products that do not use these compounds, we need to learn to read labels and find and identify products that are safe and those that are not.

DIET SODAS AND OBESITY – IS THERE A CORRELATION?

If you are overweight, and wishing to lose a few extra pounds – please, whatever you do – stay away from diet sodas!! Why? After a decade of research, I have to declare – stay away from diet sodas because only fat folks drink them! No kidding. I did a visual survey of a local soda fountain at a convenience store. Every large, overweight individual that came into the store, waddled over to the fountain and filled their cup with diet soda! Obviously and logically then, diet sodas must be what makes one fat! Of course, I am just making a little joke here, but there is indeed a very interesting correlation between diet sodas and obesity. It is a real paradox, how a beverage that contains no real caloric numbers is very likely one of the greatest causes of weight gain in the people that consume them; while all the time believing they are helping their bodies lose the weight. This is a very cruel hoax. The way this occurs is identical to the way MSG contributes to excessive weight gains.

Diet sodas are loaded with aspartame, which is 180 times sweeter than sugar – with zero calorie output. Ostensibly, this all sounds very wonderful – hey, one can drink a sweet drink, and not fill guilty about calories! As mentioned above, however, once it enters the intestinal tract, aspartame converts among other things to aspartate and phenylalanine, two highly excitable neurotransmitter amino acids, very similar in their chemical function and structures to MSG. These amino acids trigger a reflex in the chemistry of the brain called a "cephalic phase response", which simply means that once the brain registers "sweet" on the taste buds, the brain sends a signal to the body that it had better be prepared to accept pure energy, (sugar) from outside the body. The liver, then stops its manufacturing of sugar from the protein and starch reserves held in the body, and sends out its own chemical signature to STORE metabolic fuels such as fats that are circulating in the blood. In short, if the body tastes something sweet, yet the caloric energy associated with it is not forthcoming, the body goes into preservation mode; the fat-burning metabolism is slowed, and weight gain is the inevitable result! Often, appetite increases and larger meals are consumed as well because the body sends out the signal for more caloric intake. In essence, the false, sweet taste causes the brain to program the liver to store supplies instead of releasing and consuming supplies already held in storage. Like the old saying goes, (listen up Monsanto and Ajinomoto) – "It's not NICE to fool Mother Nature!"

But I don't want to pick on just diet sodas – any and all carbonated beverages are potentially dangerous dehydrating agents. If you wish to be a world-class athlete, any competent trainer will strongly advise you to remove carbonated beverages from your diet. The reason for this is really very simple, carbonated beverages lower the oxygen level in the blood, and inhibits the lungs from saturating the blood with oxygen molecules –therefore, athletic performance and endurance is compromised. If you don't believe this, lets take a quick look at how sodas get their fuzzy bubbles that tickle the nose and throat.

To make a sweet, syrupy drink fizz and bubble, pressurized Carbon Dioxide (CO_2) gas is injected into the drink. But how is Carbon Dioxide produced in the first place? We know that humans exhale this gas, and that plants consume it – but how is it pressurized commercially? In the USA, it is commercially produced through fermentation of glucose sugars by yeast, which produces ethyl alcohol and CO_2! Of course, when it is frozen, it forms that neat little product we call dry ice. When consumed in soft drinks, the unstable carbon molecule searches to bond with additional oxygen molecules in the blood, much like it's close gaseous cousin Carbon Monoxide (CO) does, (only to a lesser degree because CO_2 already has a second oxygen molecule bound to it.) According to the Merck Index, Carbon Monoxide is a "highly poisonous, odorless, colorless, tasteless, gas" while CO_2 is described as only a "colorless, odorless, noncombustible gas" with a "faint acid taste". How does Carbon Monoxide kill you? It simply combines with the hemoglobin in the blood to form carboxyhemoglobin, which in turn **DISRUPTS THE OXYGEN TRANSPORT AND DELIVERY THROUGHOUT THE BODY!!** It shuts down the brain eventually, and you simply go to sleep and never wake up. Quite peaceful really! While not as "highly poisonous" as its cousin CO, rest assured that CO_2 is still not exactly "highly nutritious" either, because it too disrupts the oxygen transport and delivery throughout the body – only not so quickly and not so efficiently! So why consume it? It is certainly not a natural product, and is certainly not nutritionally wholesome or beneficial whatsoever.

Could it be that we consume so much of it simply because billions of dollars have been spent by the soft drink giants to program our minds that carbonated beverages are not only desirable, but "wonderfully refreshing!" Cigarette ads in the past glamorized their product – but eventually good sense and the instinct of self-preservation won out. How long before the ill effects of carbonated beverages are similarly recognized? And just how much of this oxygen, and hydrogen-depleting beverage does the "average American" consume?

In the America of 1950, only about 13 ounces of soda were consumed per person per year. Coca-Cola, the "pause that refreshes" was just getting a foothold in the baby-boom generation, and the competition was just getting started with their specific "secret formulas". At the start of this new millennium, the beverage industry proudly reports that the per-capita consumption of carbonated beverages is 52.1 gallons per year. This means that every man, woman, and child in this great country consumes approximately one gallon of soda every week! Incredibly, eighty-four percent of all sodas consumed belong to only 2 companies (Coca-Cola 48.2% and Pepsi 35.9%). These giants are currently engaged in an incredible bidding war to control the exclusive marketing rights for their products on our college and university campuses. I submit this is being done to establish "brand loyalty" (taste preference) among young adults. Of course, the major universities are not going to turn away millions of dollars in "free" money, especially if it only entails allowing just one brand of soda machines in their dorms, cafeterias, and class halls. Never mind that lack of oxygenation in the brain dulls the senses and

IQ's of their students – after all is said and done, it really is apparently ALL ABOUT MONEY! Once again, Big Business Buries the Truth!

Of course, the vast majority of sodas consumed on these campuses (with the sole exception of LDS owned BYU) are laced with a drug called caffeine, which is proven to be addictive. A recent survey of students at the campus of Penn State University revealed that many students drink up to 14 cans of caffeinated sodas every day. One girl declared that she had consumed 37 Cokes in just two days! Many students admitted that they did not feel they could live without these soft drinks. If deprived of them, such victims would quickly develop withdrawal symptoms, very similar to withdrawal symptoms from other, albeit illegal, drugs. Please, I am confused, how does our western society spell H-Y-P-O-C-R-I-S-Y?? On one hand, government officials today demonize an all-natural herb of the field called hemp that many of the founding fathers of this country cultivated and consumed, (the U.S. Constitution and Declaration of Independence were written on paper made from the Hemp plant), imprisoning millions of peace-loving individuals in their massive "war on drugs", while at the same time encouraging and covering up the toxicity and deadly poison of chemical additives such as sodium fluoride, MSG, and aspartame. Big Business Buries the Truth. How very sad!

But to avoid a lawsuit for impugning their products, let me try and redeem myself and tell you a number of things that Coke (or any other similar cola product) is really very good for.

1. In many American states, the highway patrol vehicles are outfitted with two 3-liter bottles of Coke. The reason: to remove blood from the highway after a car accident! Coke does amazing things to protein molecules.

2. A really neat science fair project : Put a 2 inch-thick T-bone steak in a bowl of Coke, and only the bone will remain after 48 hours. Question to be answered, you future scientists of America: Where did the meat protein go, and WHY?

3. Toilet cleaner: Pour a can of Coke into the toilet bowl, and let the "real thing" sit for one hour, then flush away. The citric acid in the Coke removes even the most "stubborn stains" from your priceless china!

4. Remove rust spots from your chrome car bumpers and hub caps: Simply rub the bumper and hub caps with a crumbled up piece of aluminum foil dipped in Coke.

5. To clean corrosion from your car battery terminals: Pour a half a can of Coke over the terminals – the corrosion just bubbles away like magic.

6. To loosen a rusted bolt: Simply apply a cloth soaked in Coke to the rusted bolt for a few minutes. This works much better than WD-40!

7. To bake an extremely moist ham, chicken, turkey or roast: Empty a can of Coke into the baking pan, wrap the meat in aluminum foil, and bake. Thirty minutes before the meat is finished cooking, remove the foil and allow the drippings to mix with the Coke. This makes a really incredible gravy, and the heat releases the CO_2.

8. To remove grease from clothes: Empty a can of coke into a load of greasy clothes, add detergent, and run through a regular cycle. It will also clean road haze and grime from your car's windshield very effectively. Coke is fantastic for helping to loosen and remove grease stains!

Why are certain soft drinks so effective as a protein dissolver and cleaner? Simply because the active ingredient in them is phosphoric acid which has a pH of around 2.8. Phosphoric acid will dissolve a nail in about 4 days, and when consumed will absolutely leach calcium from bones and is a major contributor to osteoporosis. Did you also know that Coke distributors have been using their product to clean the engines of their trucks for over 20 years? Now the big question: would you rather have a glass of cold, pure, steam-distilled water, or a nice cold Coke?

In conclusion, the story of American Home Products (AHP) is continuing to be written. For whatever reason, in 2003 AHP decided to change its corporate name. It is now known as Wyeth Inc. The results of the Fen-Phen tragedy seem to be fading from the public consciousness. (Except for the family and friends of those who are bedridden because their hearts are permanently damaged that is, and are forced to consume Wyeth's prescription heart medications for the rest of their days.) But now Wyeth/AHP is poised for yet another financial windfall at the expense of the American public. They have developed a marvelous new flu vaccine that is inhaled directly into the nasal passages. Fantastic News! No more shots!

Called FluMist®, it is designed to replace the injected annual flu shots that millions of Americans have been brainwashed into believing they MUST have to keep from getting sick. Last "flu season" (2003-2004) was a classic example of media manipulation of the public psyche. Remember if your MSG/Aspartame/Fluoride depressed brain will let you, by some remarkable twist of fate, America came up critically short on flu vaccines. The injectable cultures somehow became contaminated. How very terrible and inconvenient! Many gullible TV viewers became panicked.

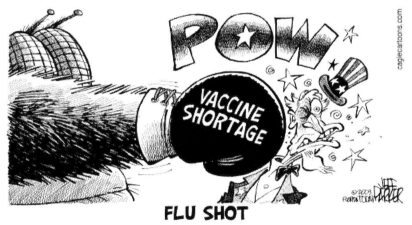

To make matters even scarier for the young and elderly, soon afterwards every TV channel was trumpeting that this year's flu strain "was particularly virulent" and lucky us, Wyeth's FluMist was the only viable option. But you had better see your doctor quickly, because "supplies were limited". Wyeth Inc. (formerly AHP) was portrayed as a knight in shining armor riding a white horse to the rescue. Hundreds of Millions of profits were generated in very short order.

Watch for AMH/Wyeth's FluMist® to quickly become the immunization of choice. Nobody likes injections and those nasty needles after all.

But guess what? FluMist® is not only loaded with Influenza bacteria, but contains high levels of MSG as well. That's right, folks. MSG, the "Essence of Taste" is added to FluMist®! At a whopping .47 MG per dose![ix] Is it there to make the dead bacteria taste better to all of the massive amounts of taste buds in our noses? What's going on?!

Conclusions: Let's see. Here is the same lab previously called American Home Products Inc. that utilized MSG to create obese rodents, in order to test their weight loss drug Fen-Phen. Now they have changed their corporate name to Wyeth and are adding the same chemical to their innovative flu vaccine!!

Clearly MSG is even more detrimental to brain neurons when consumed in the nasal passages where the blood/brain barrier is easily crossed.[x] As a nutritionist, I see nothing but villainy at work here. Think not? Ask any cocaine addict which is the most efficient way to ingest cocaine? Add it to soup and sip it? Or is it better to introduce it directly to the brain via the nasal passages? Ditto with MSG. It is proven to be bad enough when eaten and absorbed through the intestinal tract into the bloodstream. Unless one has suffered some sort of trauma to one's head, the blood/brain barrier has likely kept the drug from causing immediate major frontal lobe damage to people who are not overly sensitized. But, disguised as a harmless influenza vaccine – what damage is MSG poised to wreak now? Once again, Big Business Buries the Truth.

In Japan, Secret Assassins are called Ninja.   Ajinomoto Inc. perhaps should be renamed Ninjanomoto Inc. (meaning in English the Secret Assassin of Taste). If MSG is not a "Secret Assassin" I don't know what is!

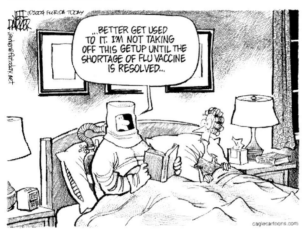

---

[i] Aninomoto Inc. News Release, May 14, 2004 – 1.039.05 Trillion Yen in NET Sales announced for fiscal year ended March 31, 2004 . www.ajinomoto.com.

[ii] Ibid

[iii] Ibid, page 8

[iv] Ibid, page 5

[v] International Diabetes Federation website 222.idf.org/home

[vi] http://www.nationmaster.com/graph-T/mor_cer_inf

[vii] http://www.nationmaster.com/country/ja/Top-Rankings

[viii] Ibid

[ix] FluMist® Package Insert (circular) page 2. http://www.flumist.com/pdf/prescribinginfo.pdf

[x] Blaylock, Dr. Russell, Excitotoxins:The Taste that Kills, Health Press, Santa Fe, 1997. Page 42

Chapter 4

The Verdict

It is proof of a base and low mind for one to wish to think with the masses or majority, merely because the majority is the majority. Truth does not change because it is, or is not, believed by a majority of the people.
- Giordano Bruno

The whole history of science has been the gradual realization that events do not happen in an arbitrary manner, but that they reflect a certain underlying order, which may or may not be divinely inspired.
- Stephen W. Hawking

On the morning of September 11, 2001, I turned on the television and was greeted with horrific news and "live" footage on virtually every cable TV channel. An undisclosed number of commercial jetliners had been hijacked and flown into select targets in New York and Washington DC. Every news channel presented the story from every possible angle. We were given the entire picture of the infamous terrorists attempting to destroy America. It seemed that our government wanted us to live in fear and trembling – and to look suspiciously at every olive-skinned man or woman of Middle Eastern descent. America, we were told, is now at war. Over 3,000 innocent American citizens were dead. Someone is responsible, and somebody has to pay.

As tragic as the events of September 11, 2001 were, what would rightfully be the levels of public outcry, or even abject panic-stricken terror in the streets of America, if the scenario of September 11 was repeated each and every day of the week? What would happen if a sinister and hidden enemy took over 3,000 innocent American lives every single day of every typical workweek? What would happen if 15,000 Americans were to die each and every week across the length and breadth of America, not just in New York City? What would happen if the grisly death toll actually surpassed the 800,000 mark for the year, and included victims from all walks of life – babies, toddlers, students, wives and mothers, husbands and fathers, healthy and productive blue and white collar professionals, as well as grandparents and those with disabilities? Would the mainstream media ignore the story, or would it merit at least a 10-minute blip on the CBS Evening News?

Well, according to a recent report, over 15,000 Americans are in fact being massacred each week across America, and amazingly, not much if anything is being reported about it. You see, the victims did not die and are not yet dying at the hands of Osama Bin Laden, Al Quaeda, or the Taliban. But unfortunately, they are just as dead, and their deaths are no less tragic. Many of them are in the prime of their lives. But unlike victims of international terrorism, the victims are massacred by the very system that has become the very backbone of American society. You see, they were needlessly killed by modern medicine – specifically by errors made by their health care practitioners and/or hospital staffs. According to the incredibly well documented report entitled "Death by Medicine", 783,936 innocent Americans died at the hands of the medical cartel in the year 2001. Let's be clear on this. These people did not die of a problematic disease such as cancer, heart disease, stroke or diabetes. ***They***

died directly because of errors made in the course of receiving routine medical treatment procedures. [i]

The problem we all face is in determining the exact number of treatment procedure errors resulting in death that are tied to not only MSG induced obesity, but to obesity related disabilities such as diabetes and heart disease. While not being able to be specific, common sense tells us that the numbers are indeed significant.

The following is a true story, however the name has been changed to respect the family's privacy. The exact details of the story may be slightly different, but it appears the same tale can be retold in every town, city and state in America.

John was born in 1958 and grew up in a small town in Nevada. He was an only child. His parents owned the local grocery store, and made a good income. John was a great sports fan as a youngster, and grew into a solid participant in his teen years. It didn't matter what sport – baseball in the summer, football in the fall, and basketball in the winter. He always had the very best equipment, and seemed to be able to showcase his skills, even though his physical stature was not exactly ideal. He was always a bit on the pudgy side. Because his family owned a grocery store, John was never at a loss for processed snack foods. When I would visit him to watch a football, basketball, or baseball game on his huge color TV – I was amazed at the CASES of potato chips, twinkies, and other junk foods piled around his bedroom and family room. Wow, John really had it made, or so I thought. How fortunate to have so many great and tasty snacks at his fingertips. Everyone in our school wished they could be as lucky as John, and to have such neat-o parents.

Looking back years later, John seemed to have peaked quite early in his high school sports career. He held a starting position on the varsity football, baseball, and basketball teams as a sophomore – but his stats and abilities actually decreased in his Junior and Senior seasons. At age 17, in the middle of his junior year, John got sick. He was diagnosed with Diabetes and had to give himself insulin injections. Nobody ever told him to eliminate or cut back on the Hostess Cup Cakes and Ding Dongs, nor to limit his soft drinks. His disease was in no way related to his diet – that was never even considered. There was absolutely no way that the MSG in the myriad of processed foods he consumed daily had anything at all to do with his failing pancreas.

Five years out of high school, at only 24 years of age, John underwent routine surgery to relieve a diabetes related circulation problem with his leg. No one knows exactly what happened, but John never made it out of the hospital. The family only said that there had been "complications" with the surgical procedure. John became a statistic – a statistic that is outlined so soberly in the report 'Death by Medicine'. According to that report, there were nearly 800,000 "complications" that led to similarly untimely deaths in 2001, just like my friend John 21 years ago.

How many millions of young people like John have lost their dreams, their health, and then their lives by ignorantly consuming the food-borne toxins MSG and Aspartame over the last 30 years? How many more lives will be shattered in the next 30 years? Can we make a conscience decision to "just say NO" to flavor enhancing drugs like MSG and Aspartame that have conclusively been shown to be causative factors in many debilitating disease conditions?

In a very real sense, each and every consumer in America is sitting on the massive jury entitled Public Opinion. You are being asked to judge this case and render a verdict, or at the very least propose an indictment. This is a mass murder trial, and the defendants have heretofore escaped responsibility.

You may render your verdict either by secret ballot or by public voice vote – it makes little difference. You see, you cast your ballot every day by refusing to purchase and/or consume items that have any form of MSG or Aspartame added to it. You cast your ballot and render your verdict by sharing this book with your friends and family. You cast your ballot and render your verdict by intelligently asking your hospital and/or health clinic why they administer IV solutions and immunizations with the known excitotoxin MSG placed in it. You cast your ballot and render your verdict by refusing to enrich the food and drug industry with your hard earned dollars to pay for any product that endangers your health and well-being.

You see, only in the elimination of, or at least substantially reducing the profit potential of such toxic substances will meaningful reforms ever be realized. Clearly, the Food and Drug Administration is not interested in protecting the people, only the pocketbooks of the medical and pharmaceutical cartel. So we must take matters into our own hands, and simply refuse to be victimized on minute longer!!

It is as simple as that. I, for one, have rendered my verdict. Guilty as charged – and as of this very minute, no more MSG and no more Aspartame will be knowingly purchased at my home or office.

---

[i] Gary Null PhD, et.al. ***Death by Medicine***, Report released in 2002, New York.

Chapter 5

The Accomplices

The birth of a man is the birth of his sorrow. The longer he lives, the more stupid he becomes, because his anxiety to avoid unavoidable death becomes more and more acute. What bitterness! He lives for what is always out of reach! His thirst for survival in the future makes him incapable of living in the present.
- Chang-Tzu

May 24, 1974 was a beautiful spring day in New York City. It started out like any other day for little William Kennerly. The precocious three year old loved his toy trucks and adored his mother. He didn't really object when she told him that she was going to take him to see a special doctor, a doctor that wanted to look at his teeth to make sure they were healthy. He could always come back home and play with his toys later.

William was happy to go downtown with Mommy. It was such a beautiful day, and he was smiling widely as he entered the Brownsville Dental Health Center in Brooklyn. William's very first dental checkup went very well, and Mrs. Kennerly was probably all smiles also when Dr. George told her that William didn't have a single cavity. He then informed her that to keep it that way, William should have a fluoride treatment. Of course, Mrs. Kennerly didn't give it a second thought, after all – Dr. George was a well-trained professional. He surely wouldn't do anything to harm little William.

Mrs. Kennerly sat and talked with Mrs. Cohen, Dr. George's dental hygienist as she proceeded to swab concentrated sodium fluoride gel over little William's small baby teeth. After thoroughly coating each tooth, Mrs. Cohen was interrupted by a question from a co-worker just as she handed William a cup of water. She didn't tell him that he should only rinse and spit the water out, so William did what most 3-year-old boys would do, he drank it right down.

Within seconds, little William was no longer smiling and happy. He started vomiting, crying, and sweating profusely while complaining in a whining voice that his head ached. When he tried to stand up, he fell over from the dizziness. Only 5 hours later, despite emergency medical treatment, little William slipped into a coma, and died. His little toy trucks were never played with again, and everyone surely missed his infectious smile.

Four and half years later, the New York Times printed the following headline: "$750,000 Given in Child's Death in Fluoride Case: Boy, 3, Was in City Clinic for Routine Cleaning".[i]

I remember this case very well. I was living in Albany, New York at the time, serving a two-year mission for my church. The details of this tragic case was discussed a number of times over dinner with different members of the local church congregation. Everyone we discussed this with had begun to question how safe fluoride really was. If it was indeed toxic, we reasoned that surely there would be some sort of warning on our toothpaste tubes, wouldn't there?

Because of the debate triggered by the death of little William Kennerly, (and hundreds of other pre-schoolers that largely went unreported), the FDA today requires fluoride toothpastes to carry a standard warning on their labels stating "if more than a pea sized amount of the toothpaste is swallowed, contact a POISON CONTROL CENTER IMMEDIATELY."

Thirty years later, however, nothing much has changed.   In dentist's chairs all over America, "hygienists" continue to swab a highly poisonous gel all over the inside of our young children's mouth. A gel, mind you, that is 20 times more poisonous than toothpaste, toothpaste that itself is so very toxic it is forced to carry one of the strongest consumer warnings of all U.S. consumer products on its labels. A consumer warning that is even stronger than tobacco products.

Of course, our children are strongly cautioned not to swallow this highly poisonous gel, but that 5-minute wait while the gel does its work can often seem like a lifetime to a young toddler or preschooler. What many parents do not realize is that during that 5-minute "treatment" the mouth is absorbing one of the most toxic poisons on the planet directly into their child's bloodstream. They do not realize that the mucous membranes located inside the mouth work like very efficient sponges, absorbing substances placed within the mouth very rapidly. This is especially true directly under the tongue. Applying a chemical under the tongue is called sublingual application, and is almost as quick and efficient as a direct hypodermic injection.

If you are at high risk for a heart attack, your doctor may prescribe nitroglycerin tablets for you to carry with you at all times. If your chest begins to ache, and you believe you are beginning a heart attack, simply put one of those small nitro pills under your tongue. It will enter the bloodstream immediately, and could probably save your life. What insanity would force a loving parent to place a deadly substance that is commonly used as rat and cockroach poison inside their child's mouth, for even one second, let alone 5 minutes? What incredible foolishness would cause American school districts to pass out sodium fluoride tablets for the students to chew and swallow?

The Merck Index, Volume 13, 2001 tells biochemists that Sodium Fluoride (NaFL) is: "Cubic or tetragonal crystals (NaCl Lattice) – **_Poisonous!_** ----- Sodium Fluoride sold as household *insecticide* must be tinted Nile Blue. LD50 orally in rats: 0.18 g/kg (remember the toxicity of MSG? – the author) **Caution:** Potential symptoms of overexposure by ingestion are salty or soapy taste; salivation, nausea, abdominal pain, vomiting, diarrhea; dehydration, thirst; sweating; stiff spine; muscle weakness, tremors; CNS depression; shock; arrhythmia. Potential symptoms of chronic ingestion are mottling of tooth enamel; osteosclerosis, calcification of ligaments of ribs and pelvis. USE: As insecticide, particularly for roaches and ants; in other pesticide formulations, (rat poison), constituent of vitreous enamel and glass mixes; as a steel degassing agent; in electroplating; in fluxes; in the fluoridation of drinking water; for disinfecting fermentation apparatus in breweries and distilleries; preserving wood, pastes and mucilage; manuf. Of coated paper; frosting glass; in removal of HF from exhaust gases to reduce air pollution. Dental caries prophylactic."[ii]

There you have it. Notice that the least common uses for chemicals listed in the Merck are listed last. I would definitely agree! The last thing I would use the toxic chemical poison Sodium Fluoride for is preventative measures (prophylactic) for tooth cavities (dental caries) by applying this poison inside my mouth! If given the choice, I would most definitely prefer a simple tooth cavity over the slow death and chronic illness caused from systematically ingesting such a highly toxic poison, wouldn't you?

Allow me to put this into perspective please. 0.18 of a gram is equal to roughly 0.00635 of an ounce. This would barely cover the head of a pin, yet if ingested orally by a rat, this miniscule amount would kill it. No wonder that the primary historical use for Sodium Fluoride is as the "active ingredient" in various insecticides and vermin poisons. What lunacy is this to ingest a highly toxic poison in the false hope of preventing cavities??

Consider if you will, that in a few of these United States, you can still receive the death penalty upon conviction of premeditated murder. The much preferred "humane" method of execution is death by lethal injection. The U.S. penal system provides the chemical poison to inject. It needs to be very quick and efficient, or the ACLU would scream even louder. Everyone, (except perhaps the family of the deceased victim) agrees there is no real need to make the convicted murderer suffer needlessly. So the system searched out the most efficient and humane poison available. I am confident that the penal officials considered Sodium Fluoride very long and very hard. It likely made their very short list. You see, there simply are not too many chemical poisons available on planet earth that is more efficient and deadly ounce for ounce than sodium fluoride, the active ingredient in your toddler's tube of "Blue's Clues" berry flavored toothpaste. Instead of sodium fluoride, however, the benevolent executioners decided on a chemically hybridized form of curare, the poison used by South American Indians to coat the tips of their poisoned arrows. Called Intocostrin, this substance affects the neuromuscular system first, then within minutes robs the brain of oxygen. The brain shuts down, the victim goes to sleep, and death occurs within a few short minutes. As efficient as this designer drug of the executioner is, it is only slightly more toxic than Sodium Fluoride, having a lethal dosage (LD) of just over .10 g/kg.

THE NATIONAL 'SCANDAL' THAT IS CALLED FLOURIDE

It needs to be stated that the substance referred to as "fluoride" is a misnomer. There simply is no such substance listed in the periodic chart of the elements, or in the prestigious CRC handbook, or even in the sacred bible of the pharmaceutical industry – the illustrious Merck Index. Instead, we find a GAS called Fluorine – and from the use of this gas in various industries such as aluminum manufacturing and the nuclear industry –certain toxic byproducts are created which have "captured" fluorine molecules. One such toxic, poisonous manufacturing "byproduct" is called sodium fluoride. Sodium fluoride is found in the Merck Index and the CRC handbook. Again, according to the Merck Index it is primarily used as rat and cockroach poison and is also the active ingredient in most toothpastes and as an "additive to drinking water". But sadly, there is much more to this sordid tale.

Did you know that sodium fluoride is also one of the basic ingredients in both PROZAC (Fluoxetene Hydrochloride) and Sarin Nerve Gas (Isopropyl-Methyl-Phosphoryl FLUORIDE) – (Yes, folks the same Sarin Nerve Gas that terrorists released a decade ago on a crowded Japanese subway train!). Let me repeat: the truth the American public needs to understand is the fact that sodium fluoride is nothing more (or less) than a hazardous, toxic waste by-product of the nuclear and aluminum industries. In addition to being the primary ingredient in rat and cockroach poisons, it is also a main ingredient in anesthetic, hypnotic, and psychiatric drugs as well as military NERVE GAS! Why, oh why then is it allowed by the FDA to be added to the toothpastes and drinking water of the American people?

Our benevolent government and the news media have declared sodium fluoride to be a "substance that helps prevent cavities." Let me again declare the solemn truth! Sodium fluoride is a manmade compound created as a poisonous byproduct of aluminum manufacturing and is the KEY INGREDIENT in most RAT POISONS!! You will never hear the news media or your dentist tell you "sodium fluoride is good for your teeth", for the lawsuit would be massive; but yet, when you buy toothpaste with so-called "fluoride" in it you need to look at the fine print on the label. It does not say "fluoride", but rather says sodium fluoride or "stannous fluoride" (another harmful, toxic compound – not a natural element.) Your dentist can legally tell you that "fluoride" is good for your teeth, because technically there is no such substance. It is like telling you the "tooth fairy" will protect your teeth from cavities, it is a fictional character that simply does not exist! The sad truth is that your professional dentist simply does not know any better! He doesn't know and understand the following true history.

Historically, sodium fluoride was quite expensive for the worlds' premier chemical companies to dispose of. In the decade of the 50's, Alcoa and the entire aluminum industry, with a vast overabundance of the toxic waste chemical named NaFl, SOMEHOW sold the FDA and our government on the insane (but highly profitable) idea of buying this poison at a 20,000% markup and then injecting it into our water supply as well as into the nation's toothpastes and dental gels. Yes that's correct, folks – a 20,000% markup.

Consider also that when sodium fluoride is injected into our drinking water, its level is approximately 1 part-per-million (ppm). However, since we only drink ½ of one percent (.005%) of the total water supply, this hazardous chemical literally "goes down the drain" and voila – the chemical industry has not only a free hazardous waste disposal system, but we have also PAID them handsomely for solving their disposal problem!! Once again Big Business Buries the Truth.

The Truth is that the Aluminum Company of America (ALCOA) became enormously wealthy during the roaring 20's. It's founder and president was a gentleman named Andrew Mellon. His wealth and influence was a great asset to Washington politicians and presidential hopefuls. In 1928, Mellon was appointed the Treasury Secretary for the United States government. He held that position until the mid 1930's. Secretary Mellon's fiscal policies helped plunge American into the Great Depression, and made the U.S. Treasury subservient to the private Federal Reserve banks. Mellon was also in control of a new bureaucracy named the U.S. Public Health Service (USPHS). How very convenient. He saw a golden opportunity to solve ALCOA's number one problem, disposing of his toxic poisonous mountains of sodium fluoride. He wondered if he could possibly pull off the big con. Could his mountains of sodium fluoride possibly be packaged as a "beneficial health additive"?

In 1928, a man named Frederick McKay observed something a bit unusual. He found that teeth that had been exposed to sodium fluoride developed a sort of "mottling" effect. He wondered in a public letter to Mr. Melling if this "mottling" could prevent the formation of cavities.[iii] He petitioned Mr. Mellon and Mellon's USPHS to commission him to conduct a study on the subject.

Then in 1931, Mellon commissioned his friend, H. Trendley Dean of the USPHS to study the nation's water supplies. Dean determined that as sodium fluoride levels increased in water, so did the amount of fluorosis on teeth. His research continued, and in the late 1930's, he published completely skewed and unscientifically supported data showing that at a concentration of 1 part per million, sodium fluoride "produced a minimal amount of dental fluorisis and resulted in the reduction of tooth decay." [iv]

When word of what Mellon was attempting reached the ears of the American Dental Association and the American Medical Association, they immediately came out in strong vocal and written opposition to the moronic notion of a well-known poison such as sodium fluoride being considered as a health additive. The editorial board of the prestigious Journal of the American Medical Association published the following facts: *'Fluorides are general protoplasmic poisons ------the sources of fluorine intoxication are drinking water containing 1 part per million or more of fluorine--------another source of fluorine intoxication is from the fluorides used in the smelting of many metals, such as steel and aluminum.'[v]* Notice that the AMA specifically states "fluoride intoxication" occurs in 1 ppm levels in water, the exact amount that is today recommended by governmental health agencies to be added to water supplies.

The American Dental Association in their Journal quickly echoed the AMA's stand. It declared: *"We do know the use of drinking water containing as little as 1.2 to 3.0 parts per million of fluorine will cause such developmental disturbances in bones as osteosclerosis, spondylosis and osteopetrosis, as well as goiter, and we cannot afford to run the risk of producing such serious systemic disturbances in applying what is at present a doubtful procedure intended to prevent development or dental disfigurements among children." –Journal of the American Dental Association.* [vi] What made the ADA reverse its stand against sodium fluoride, and enthusiastically embrace this poison just a decade later? Political pressures and Big Money interests did the job. Yet another example of Big Business Buries the Truth.

Andrew Mellon, chemical industrialist and billionaire, the corporate force behind the federal reserve system and fluoridation, died under a cloud in 1937. His name had been disgraced as the corrupt U.S. Treasurer whose short-sighted cronyism helped start the Great Depression. Though he was dead, however, his toxic legacy continued to live on thanks to his hand-picked successors at ALCOA. Specifically a shrewd attorney named Oscar Ewing finished the job, and successfully brainwashed America to consume a toxic waste product called sodium fluoride and PAY to do it.

Ewing, as legal counsel for ALCOA, was paid the paltry sum of $750,000 dollars a year in the early 1940's (which is the equivalent of over $8 million in 2005 dollars). In 1944, he inexplicably left his position at ALCOA to take an incredibly dramatic pay cut and became the Federal Security Administrator. In 1944, this bureaucratic position was directly over the United States Public Health Service. [vii] FSA Chief Ewing then hired the nephew of Sigmund Frued, a man named Edward Bernays, to work in his office. Bernays authored a book in 1928 entitled ***Propaganda!*** The book outlined in precise detail how to successfully manipulate public opinion to achieve a desired result. In essence, it was the official handbook of how to produce a favorable "Problem, Reaction, and Solution" scenario. Under Bernay's tutelage, Oscar Ewing successfully manipulated popular opinion, and made the AMA and ADA opponents of fluoridation look like "crackpots and right wing loonies". [viii] Little has changed since then.

Ewing's fluoridation propaganda juggernaut began its frontal assault on America in 1945. Grand Rapids Michigan became the first American community to add sodium fluoride to its culinary water. Within two years, six more U.S. cities and 87 small towns decided to add sodium fluoride to their water tanks. They had bought into Bernay's mindless propaganda after reading full-page advertisements in publications such as the Journal of American Water Works Association proclaiming: ***"ALCOA sodium fluoride is particularly suitable for the fluoridation of water supplies............If your community is fluoridating its water supply – or is considering doing so – let us show you how ALCOA sodium fluoride can do the job for you."***[ix] Once a sizable number of municipalities began adding this toxin, the floodgates were opened. They could not reverse course and risk admitting any liabilities. The Propaganda only intensified. In 1950, the American Dental Association accepted large grants from ALCOA, and together with Ewing's United States

Public Health Service issued a joint endorsement extolling the "safety and benefits" of water fluoridation. This was done without any scientific data and studies to back up their declarations. Big Business successfully Buried the Truth. As of the year 2005, concerning fluoride poisons, it is still to this day largely buried 6 feet under.

Keep in mind that this was at a time when the American public was reveling in the successful conclusion of WWII. Anything Truman and/or General Eisenhower's government declared was perceived to be the gospel truth, and did not need to be challenged. The USPHS then started promoting fluoridation nationwide. The propaganda machine entered new heights and breadth.

In 1951, Frank Bull, the Director of Dental Education for the Wisconsin State Board of Health gave a speech at the Washington Conference of State Dental Directors that reflected the half-truth of Ewing and Bernay concerning how to "sell professionals" on promoting ALCOA's sodium fluoride. He declared: *"Now in regard to toxicity.....the term "adding sodium fluoride" We NEVER DO THAT! Sodium fluoride is rat poison. You add fluorides. Never mind that sodium fluoride business.....if it is a fact that some individuals are against fluoridation, you have just got to knock their objections down. The question of toxicity is on the same order. Lay off it altogether. Just pass it over. 'We know there is absolutely no effect other than reducing tooth decay,' you say and go on."* [x] This "Bull" must have been exceptionally deep, because to this day, the American Dental Association website (*www.ada.org*) sticks to Bull's 1951 directives, declaring that even though children's teeth may be permanently scarred with fluorosis (declared by the 1944 ADA to be "Permanent Disfigurement") it is worth the risk to reduce cavities. In the mid 50's, it became posh and fashionable to "brush the teeth" with a sodium fluoride toothpaste. America has never looked back.

Today, the truth is that over 80% of children in communities with sodium- fluoridated water, combined with sodium-fluoridated toothpaste use, have teeth visibly discolored by the toxic effect of fluoride. [xi] Compare that rate with the 0% rate in communities with no fluoride in their drinking water. Moreover, the Bull put out in the pattern prescribed by Bernay's propaganda manual is yet being employed. Concerned community activists today are being told that the form of fluoride is not the toxic "sodium fluoride" molecule, but the benign and wonderful "Hydrogen-based fluoride." Please do not be fooled by the bull. There is only one manufacturer of water fluoridation chemicals – and that is ALCOA or one of its wholly owned subsidiaries. It may be labeled as something different, but rest assured, the source is always the toxic waste product sodium fluoride produced by ALCOA's aluminum factory smoke stacks. Never forget that Big Business Buries the Truth, often by disguising it in slick advertisements and propaganda. ALCOA has made TRILLIONS of dollars on this scam, and it shows no signs of slowing down.

Aside from dental fluorosis, there are much more important issues associated with fluoridation. Nobody really knows how sodium fluoride toxins combine with monosodium glutamate or aspartame in the brain. Independent scientific evidence over the past 50 plus years has shown that sodium fluoride, like MSG and Aspartame shortens our life span, promotes various cancers and mental disturbances, and most importantly, makes humans stupid, docile, and subservient, all in one neat little package. There is increasing evidence that aluminum in the brain, along with MSG and Aspartame, is a causative factor in Alzheimer's Disease. Evidence points towards sodium fluoride's strong affinity to bond with aluminum (remember it is a byproduct of aluminum manufacturing) and also it has the ability to "trick" the blood-brain barrier by imitating the hydrogen ion thus allowing this chemical access to brain tissue by crossing the blood-brain barrier.[xii]

Honest scientists who have attempted to blow the whistle on ALCOA's mega-bucks sodium fluoride propaganda campaign have consistently been given a large dose of professional "black-balling". As a result, their valid points disputing the current corporate vested interests never have received the ink they deserve in the national press. Just follow the money to find the "control" and you will find prominent American families to be prominent players in the scandal. In 1952 a slick PR campaign rammed the concept of fluoridation through our Public Health departments and various dental organizations. This slick campaign was more akin to a highly emotional "beer salesman convention" instead of the objective, scientifically researched program that it should have been. It has continued in the same vein right up to the present day – and now sodium fluoride use has now become "usual and customary", as has Aspartame and MSG.

To illustrate the emotional vs. the scientific nature of this issue, just look at the response given by people (perhaps yourself included?) when the subject of fluoridation comes up. You need to ask yourself,

"Is this particular response based on EMOTIONS born of TRADITION, or is it truly unbiased and based instead on thoroughly researched objectivity?" There is a tremendous amount of emotional, highly unscientific "know-it-all" emotions attached to the topic of sodium fluoride usage. I personally have yet to find even ONE objective, double blind study that even remotely links sodium fluoride to healthy teeth at ANY AGE. Instead, I hear and read such mindless rhetoric as "9 out of 10 DENTISTS recommend 'fluoride' toothpaste" etc. etc. etc. Let me reiterate: truly independent (unattached to moneyed vested interest groups) scientists who've spent a large portion of their lives studying and working with this subject have been hit with a surprising amount of unfair character assassinations from strong vested-interest groups who reap grand profits from the public's ignorance as well as from the public's illnesses. Just follow the money! Big Business Buries the Truth.

There are reportedly more than 16 million Americans with diabetes, and thanks to MSG, that number is skyrocketing every year. If it is true that diabetics drink more liquids than other people, then according to the Physicians Desk Reference these 16 million people are at much higher risk drinking fluoridated water because they will receive a much deadlier dose because of their need for higher than normal water consumption.

Kidney disease, by definition, lowers the efficiency of the kidneys, which of course is the primary bodily function in which fluoride (or any other toxic chemical) is eliminated from the body. Does it not make sense that these people shouldn't drink fluoridated water at all? Cases are on record (Annapolis, Maryland, 1979) where ill kidney patients on dialysis machines died because they ingested relatively small amounts of SODIUM FLUORIDE from unwittingly drinking the fluoridated city water supply![xiii] Will adequate warnings be given to people with weak kidneys, or will the real cause of such deaths be 'covered up' in the name of 'domestic tranquility'?

Concerning the "practice" of putting sodium fluoride into drinking water, where did this insanity begin and WHO tried it first? From personal research, I was shocked and dismayed to find out that the Nazis were the first to intentionally place sodium fluoride into drinking water supplies. This was accomplished in the Polish ghettos and in Nazi Germany's infamous prison camps. The Gestapo you see had little concern about sodium fluoride's supposed effect on children's teeth; instead, their reason for mass-medicating water with sodium fluoride was to STERILIZE SUPPOSEDLY "INFERIOR" HUMANS and force the people in their concentration camps into calm, bovine, submission. (See for reference: "The Crime and Punishment of I.G. Farben" written by Joseph Borkin.) Kind of shocking isn't it folks!! Ah, but it gets even better.

In a book entitled The Secret Backers of Hitler, the author exposes that certain wealthy American industrialists placed tens of millions of dollars at Adolph Hitler's disposal to build and orchestrate his "Third Reich". One such wealthy industrialist was none other than Andrew Mellon. This helps us to better understand the charges leveled by certain scientists concerning ALCOA's motives, and why Mellon died under a political cloud.

The following letter was received by the Lee Foundation for Nutritional Research, Milwaukee Wisconsin, on 2 October 1954, from a research chemist by the name of Charles Perkins. He writes:

"I have your letter of September 29 asking for further documentation regarding a statement made in my book, "The Truth about Water Fluoridation", to the effect that the idea of water fluoridation was brought to England from Russia by the Russian Communist Kreminoff. In the 1930's Hitler and the German Nazis envisioned a world to be dominated and controlled by a Nazi philosophy of pan-Germanism. The German chemists worked out a very ingenious and far-reaching plan of mass-control which was submitted to and adopted by the German General Staff. This plan was to control the population in any given area through mass medication of drinking water supplies. By this method they could control the population in whole areas, reduce population by water medication that would produce sterility in women, and so on. In this scheme of mass-control, sodium fluoride occupied a prominent place.

"Repeated doses of infinitesimal amounts of fluoride will in time reduce an individual's power to resist domination, by slowly poisoning and narcotizing a certain area of the brain, thus making him submissive to the will of those who wish to govern him. [A convenient and cost-effective light lobotomy? --- Ott].

"The real reason behind water fluoridation is not to benefit children's teeth. If this were the real reason there are many ways in which it could be done that are much easier, cheaper, and far more effective.   The real purpose behind water fluoridation is to reduce the resistance of the masses to domination and control and loss of liberty."

"When the Nazis under Hitler decided to go to Poland, both the German General Staff and the Russian General Staff exchanged scientific and military ideas, plans, and personnel, and the scheme of mass control through water medication was

seized upon by the Russian Communists because it fitted ideally into their plans to communize the world."

"I was told of this entire scheme by a German chemist who was an official of the great I.G. Farben chemical industries and was also prominent in the Nazi movement at the time. I say this with all the earnestness and sincerity of a scientist who has spent nearly 20 years' research into the chemistry, biochemistry, physiology and pathology of fluorine --- any person who drinks artificially fluorinated water for a period of one year or more will never again be the same person mentally or physically."
    Signed: CHARLES E. PERKINS, Chemist, 2 October, 1954.

Another letter needs to be quoted at length as well to help corroborate Mr. Perkin's testimony. The letter was written by a brilliant (and objectively honest) scientist named Dr. E.H. Bronner. Dr. Bronner was a nephew of the great Albert Einstein, served time in a WWII prison camp and wrote the following letter printed in the Catholic Mirror, Springfield, MA, January 1952:

"It appears that the citizens of Massachusetts are among the 'next' on the agenda of the water poisoners.

"There is a sinister network of subversive agents, Godless intellectual parasites, working in our country today whose ramifications grow more extensive, more successful and more alarming each new year and whose true objective is to demoralize, paralyze and destroy our great Republic ---- from within if they can, according to their plan --- for their own possession."

"The tragic success they have already attained in their long siege to destroy the moral fiber of American life is now one of their most potent footholds towards their own ultimate victory over us."

"Fluoridation of our community water systems can well become their most subtle weapon for our sure physical and mental deterioration. As a research chemist of established standing, I built within the past 22 years 3 American chemical plants and licensed 6 of my 53 patents. Based on my years of practical experience in the health food and chemical field, let me warn: fluoridation of drinking water is criminal insanity, sure national suicide. DON'T DO IT!!"

"Even in very small quantities, sodium fluoride is a deadly poison to which no effective antidote has been found. Every exterminator knows that it is the most effective rat-killer. Sodium Fluoride is entirely different from organic calcium-fluoro-phosphate needed by our bodies and provided by nature, in God's great providence and love, to build and strengthen our bones and our teeth. This organic calcium-fluoro-phosphate, derived from proper foods, is an edible organic salt, insoluble in water and assimilable by the human body; whereas the non-organic sodium fluoride used in fluoridating water is instant poison to the body and fully water soluble. The body refuses to assimilate it."

"Careful, bonafide laboratory experimentation by conscientious, patriotic research chemists, and actual medical experience, have both revealed that instead of preserving or promoting 'dental health', fluoridated drinking water destroys teeth before adulthood and after, by the destructive mottling and other pathological conditions it actually causes in them, and also creates many other very grave pathological conditions in the internal organisms of bodies consuming it. How then can it be called a 'health plan'? What's behind it?"

"That any so-called 'Doctors' would persuade a civilized nation to add voluntarily a deadly poison to its drinking water systems is unbelievable. It is the height of criminal insanity!"

"No wonder Hitler and Stalin fully believed and agreed from 1939 to 1941 that, quoting from both Lenin's 'Last Will' and

Hitler's Mein Kampf: *"America we shall demoralize, divide, and destroy from within."*

"Are our Civil Defense organizations and agencies awake to the perils of water poisoning by fluoridation? Its use has been recorded in other countries. Sodium Fluoride water solutions are the cheapest and most effective rat killers known to chemists: colorless, odorless, tasteless; no antidote, no remedy, no hope: Instant and complete extermination of rats."

"Fluoridation of water systems can be slow national suicide, or quick national liquidation. It is criminal insanity ------- treason!!"
Signed: Dr. E.H. Bronner, Research Chemist, Los Angeles

Apparently, the public outcry by Dr. Bronner and others precluded the sodium- fluoridation of public water systems for a season – but soon thereafter, the Food and Drug Administration allowed this deadly poison to be put in tooth "paste", and our dentists were systematically brainwashed into providing "fluoride" treatments to their many patients. Of course, today many major metropolitan areas have a minimum of 1 parts per million sodium fluoride systematically added to their water supply and more areas are seeking to add this poison every year. Add to this the fact that bottling companies (soft drinks, juices, etc.) use fluoridated water to make their products – is it any wonder that people can no longer think clearly and ask pertinent questions of their elected and ecclesiastical leaders? Is it also still a mystery why the CIA and their infamous "Operation Paper Clip" brought many top Nazi mind control scientists to America?

If you believe all of this is "just a coincidence" and the author is just a right wing conspiracy nut, please by all means go ahead and keep brushing your teeth with your sodium fluoride toothpaste and sucking on your sodium fluoridated Coke or Pepsi product to wash down your MSG laden potato chips. For you, ignorance truly is bliss and you truly will reap what you have sown.

Mothers, if your little ones are having trouble concentrating at home or in school, or have been diagnosed as "attention deficit" in addition to eliminating MSG perhaps you would be well advised to look for the culprit no further than your home medicine cabinet (your tube of toothpaste) and your friendly neighborhood school's fluoridated water fountain!!

In the United States, a manual called Pharmacopia, A Guide to Drug Information states: **"The side effects of daily ingestion of the amount of sodium fluoride found in one to two pints of fluoridated water are as follows: black tarry stools, bloody vomit, faintness, nausea, vomiting, shallow breathing, stomach cramps, pain, tremors, unusual excitement, unusual increase in saliva, watery eyes, weakness, constipation, loss of appetite, pain and aches of bones, skin rash, sores in the mouth and lips, stiffness, weight loss, white, brown, or black DISCOLORATION OF TEETH."**

Make no mistake about it, sodium fluoride reacts in the body AS A POISON. According to the 1984 issue of Clinical Toxicology, (Williams and Wilkes), it is more poisonous than lead, and only slightly less poisonous than arsenic. In 1991, the Akron Ohio Regional Poison Center reported a death following the ingestion of only 16 milligrams of sodium fluoride. In plan English, this means that $1/100^{th}$ of one ounce of sodium fluoride can kill a 10-pound child, and $1/10^{th}$ of an ounce can kill an adult. The Akron Center continued to state that a pinch of fluoride toothpaste contains up to one milligram of sodium fluoride. This means that a "family-sized" tube of toothpaste contains 199 milligrams of sodium fluoride, more than enough to kill a 25-pound child.

In a study of 43 ready-to-drink fruit juices by Dr. J.J. Stannard and co-workers, sodium fluoride concentrations in common beverages were examined. It was found that 42% of the samples had more than 1 part per million sodium fluoride. An analysis of Coke Classic bottled in Chicago showed 2.56 parts per million sodium fluoride. Diet Coke bottled in Chicago tested 2.96 parts per million sodium fluoride. Sodium Fluoride is found in virtually all soft drinks and drinks from concentrate because every major bottling plant in this country was built in a city that added sodium fluoride to its local drinking water. Funny, but under federal law – they don't have to disclose this on their label. If you want to avoid sodium fluoride, care should be taken to avoid all beverages such as soft drinks, beers, wines, and juice drinks from concentrate. Frozen concentrates or fresh, unconstituted drinks are the safest.

It seems to me that the American people have been targeted by an elite few in a most heinous manner. For some reason, certain parties appear eager to keep the grassroots not only ignorant, but also just ill enough not to be able to think coherently and rationally. I cannot understand any other explanation as to why any government would be participating in systematically poisoning its citizens.

CHLORINE – ANOTHER POISONOUS CHEMICAL

A few years ago, German swimmers visiting the U.S. as part of an international competition steadfastly refused to enter an American swimming pool because of the large chlorine content in the water. Were they correct in their belief, or were they, (as local media coverage claimed) merely paranoid "prudes"? No, I would submit that the Germans know all too well the dangers of chlorine gas. In the trenches of WWI France, they witnessed the deadly effects, but back then it was known as mustard gas, or bertholite, and it disabled and killed many a soldier on both sides of the trenches. Yep, this surely appears to be a good, wholesome chemical to add to our drinking water, swimming pools, and spas.

Following WWI, chlorine was added to culinary water systems in the U.S. ostensibly to kill bacterial pathogens in the water. What is truly amazing is the utter stupidity of such an act. Imagine, adding a known poison to one's drinking water to rid it of a less damaging pest. It is the mental equivalent of releasing a king cobra into your home to hunt and eradicate the rat you saw yesterday in your bathroom! There are better, and safer ways to take care of such problems. They are called rat-traps and ozonation!

Yes, it is true that chlorine is only added in minute quantities, but it still causes a myriad of health problems in humans when consumed. First of all, yes, chlorine kills harmful microorganisms, but when consumed in drinking water, it also kills many, if not all of the BENEFICIAL, friendly bacteria in your intestinal tract. These bacteria break down your food that you ate last night, and are critical components of digestion. They also protect the body from harmful pathogens.   In addition, these wonderful little critters manufacture important vitamins like B12 and vitamin K.   Directly because of drinking chlorinated water, chronic digestive disorders and problem skin conditions like acne, psoriasis, seborrhea and eczema are manifest. (Such disorders often clear up in rapid order by following two simple steps: 1. consuming purified distilled water, and 2. reintroducing friendly bacteria by supplementing lactobacillus acidophilus and bifidus for a couple of months.)

But of course, there is so much more to the sordid tale. For the last 3 decades, the water treatment and chemical industries have KNOWN that chlorine combines with naturally benign and harmless organic compounds present in water to form brand new chemical compounds that are toxic and carcinogenic.   These natural compounds are called humus, humic acid, and fulvic acid – terms used to describe substances that are essentially ancient compost material.   Decayed leaves and other vegetation breaks down chemically over time, and this material enters into ground water aquifers.   Once the breakdown is completed, science calls the solid substance soil humus, and the liquid by-product humic and fulvic acids.   These liquids are water soluble and readily transported into streams, waterways, lakes, and of course groundwater reservoirs. From there, of course, they enter our culinary water systems for human consumption.

The culinary water systems have a nice little name for the toxic compounds created by introducing chlorine with these normally harmless, (and in many cases health promoting) organic acids. They call these toxins DBP's or disinfection by-products, a term that makes them sound quite harmless and innocuous. However, the most common group of DBP's are called trihalomethanes (or THMs); and these bad boys are KNOWN CARCINOGENS – in other words, they cause cancer! THMs are not by any means single chemicals either, but are a whole class of compounds unto themselves that include chloroform (CHCl3), bromoform (CHBr3) dichlorobromomethane (CHCl2Br) and dibromochloromethane (CHClBR2). I know these are big mouthfuls, but most harmful chemical toxins usually are. You may have heard of chloroform. It is what the villains in countless cloak and dagger mystery movies used to put their victims instantly to sleep. Continuous and steady exposure results in death, albeit a very peaceful demise. This is why "humane" vets used chloroform extensively to "put sick pets TO SLEEP" – just a humane term for killing them peacefully. Could this be one more reason why so many Americans are 'asleep' and do not take responsibility for their own health. Are we slowly being chloroformed by our chlorinated waters?

THMs do not degrade very well and are usually stored in the fatty tissues of the body (breast, other fatty areas, mother's milk, blood, and semen). Also referred to as organochlorides, THMs can and do cause mutations by altering DNA, suppressing immune system functions, and interfering with the natural controls of cellular growth. Studies have shown they cause a high incidence of bladder and colorectal cancer in populations whose drinking water contains them. According to the U.S. News and World Report magazine, July 1991 edition: "Drinking chlorinated water may as much as double the risk of Bladder Cancer, which strikes 40,000 people a year." A study done in Canada and released in 1995 concluded that long-term drinking and bathing in chlorinated water likely causes a 34% increase in the incidence of bladder and colon cancer.[xiv] It also found that the risk increases with the length of exposure and the concentration of chlorinated by-products in the water. In those areas where the by-products of chlorination were high, the increased incidence could be higher than 60% for people who have used the water for more than 35 years. Furthermore, it may well be that it is mainly chlorine, and not cholesterol, that is the real culprit behind the high increase in heart disease in this country. (Overly heated and processed milk products also appear to be major factors as well, however).

A study in Finland followed 1,222 Helsinki businessmen considered at high risk of heart attack for 15 years. Half were put on an intensive program including dietary regulations; the other half served as a control group. After 15 years, the low-cholesterol group had FAR MORE DEATHS than the control group who ate "normally"!! Those who cut their "harmful cholesterol" had 67 deaths overall, with 34 from heart disease. The control group had less than half the overall death-rate with only 14 cardiac related deaths!![xv] Cholesterol is not the deadly killer the medical propaganda machine makes it out to be. Chlorine is much more dangerous.

The wellness secret that you must understand is that this wildly explosive increase in the incidence of cardiovascular disease and fatal heart attacks began in 1920, the same year we began chlorinating our water following the successful trial of chlorine gas on the battlefields of WW I. If I didn't know better, and didn't blindly trust our government so much, I could almost come to the conclusion that some group within our bureaucracy wishes to bilk the public trust while keeping the people less than optimally healthy. But then, if I thought such a thing I would surely be labeled a wacko conspiracy theorist, or worse – a terrorist threat as defined by the new Patriot Act because I could be "causing a panic" among the chemically controlled populace! Never mind that this heart disease explosion was ***only in those countries adding chlorine to their drinking waters!!*** For instance, cardiovascular diseases remained virtually unknown in China, Japan, Africa, and Asia. However, when Japanese citizens emigrated to Hawaii where the water was chlorinated, they suffered the exact same rate of heart attacks as Americans, even though their diets were very much identical to relatives back in Japan. Similarly, the black population in the US has the average US rate of heart attacks, but not their brothers in Africa. It is the same with inhabitants of the non-chlorinated Roseto in Pennsylvania who were free of heart attacks unless and until they moved to chlorinated water areas. Again, just coincidence? You decide for yourself – but for me, if it looks like a duck, walks like a duck, quacks like a duck, swims like a duck, and has webbed feet, feathers, and a funny shaped bill – why not just cut to the chase and call it a duck? If the federal government wishes to call it a chicken – that is their choice even though I choose to think for myself and not agree. Just don't brainwash me by propaganda and public opinion manipulation into actually believing the Emperor is really wearing clothes when he is standing in front of me stark naked, and please don't tell me that such manufactured fiction is hard fact.

In 1967 a Dr. J. Price in the U.S. performed a very decisive experiment. He added only 1/3 of a teaspoon of chlorine bleach to a liter of water for one group of 50 three-month-old chickens (cockerels). Another group of 50 chickens served as the control group. Seven months later over 95% of the chlorinated group had advanced arterioscleroses; NONE of the control group had any problem whatsoever. Dr. Price repeated his experiment many, many times – always with the exact same result. Recently even researchers funded by the EPA have confirmed arteriosclerotic-type changes in other animals as well, including primate monkeys, when exposed to chlorinated water. Here are two direct quotes from Dr. Price:

"The cause of arterioscleroses and resulting heart attacks and strokes is none other than the ubiquitous chlorine in our drinking water. Chlorine is the greatest crippler and killer of the modern times. While it prevented epidemics of one disease, it was creating another. Two decades ago, after the start of chlorinating our drinking water in 1920, the present epidemic of the heart trouble, cancer, and senility began."

Here is yet another quote from Dr. Riddle, PhD, at Kemysts Laboratory, giving the range of diseases linked to Chlorine:

"Scientific studies have linked chlorine and chlorination by-products to cancer of the bladder, liver, rectum, and colon, as well as heart disease, arteriosclerosis (hardening of the arteries), anemia, high blood pressure, and allergic reactions."

In addition, some investigations have found these chlorination by-products may also be linked to kidney and central nervous system damage. Other studies have linked them to reproductive problems, including miscarriage. A California study found a miscarriage rate of

15.7% for women who drank 5 or more glasses of water containing more than 75 ppb (parts per billion) THM, compared to a miscarriage rate of only 9.5% for women with low THM exposure.

To their credit, the EPA is continually tightening their restrictions on THMs in drinking water. However, it is truly an impossible battle to win. Once the choice was made by the government to chlorinate, we have been locked into using a poison named chlorine that creates even more and deadlier poisons with each substance it comes in contact with!!

The most recent information about chlorine's uncanny ability to combine with otherwise beneficial elements to create new poisons is even worse news. Researchers in Japan found that when the chlorine in our tap water combines with many of nature's most beneficial nutrients, it once again creates deadly cancer-causing substances. Research scientists at the National Institute of Health Sciences and Shizuoka Prefectural University made these discoveries in a joint study. They determined that natural organic substances originating from foods, including fruits, soy, and green or black tea, react when tap water is chlorinated, forming dangerous cancer causing compounds. (These particular foods were used because the study involved the Japanese diet – other foods could well react the same way!) These deadly new carcinogens have been named MX, which simply stands for "unknown mutagen". These compounds are quite similar to the THM's described above.

These studies show the shocking truth that MX is created by the reaction of chlorine with natural organic plant phytochemicals such as catechins, which are found in tea, and flavonoids, which are found in fruit. In 1997, scientists in Finland found MX to be 170 times more deadly than other known toxic by-products of chlorination, and their laboratory studies showed these substances damage the thyroid gland, and cause cancerous tumors. Little wonder why those German swimmers refused to enter a pool that was heavily chlorinated! I wonder what effect chlorine has on MSG and Aspartame in the human body?

WHAT DOES ALL OF THIS MEAN?

Until just recently, we simply didn't have good information about the actual composition of humus, humic acid, and fulvic acid. New scientific discoveries have identified and clarified their composition. These natural substances in fact contain a significant amount of nutritional phytochemical groups including hormones, sterols, fatty acids, alkaloids, polyphenols and ketones. The subgroups of these substances include but are not limited to: flavins, flavonoids, flovones, tannins, catechins, quinines, isoflavones, tocopherols, ets. I know, I know, big boring words, but they are keys to helping us unlock the mystery of mineralization and bio-chemistry, so please bear with me.

If you are fairly well educated in the field of nutrition, you may recognize that these newly discovered substances are some of the very most valuable and promising health-promoting and anti-cancer nutrients found in our foods and health supplements. For example, Coenzyme Q-10 is a quinine, vitamin B2 is a flavin, vitamin E is a tocopherol. Citrus bioflavonoids including hesperidin, quercetin, and rutin are all flavonoids – and green tea contains catechins, phenols, tannins and isofavones. Potentially all of these substances, and many more, are turned into poisons by chlorination.

Furthermore, it has been discovered that nature, in her infinite wisdom, has ensured that these phytochemicals remain intact, concentrated, and intricately combined within humic substances over thousands and even millions of years.   These humics are the extremely valuable remnants of nature's beneficial substances contained within fruits, flowers, pollen, nuts and seeds, as well as roots, stems, bark, and leaves. Even the plant based nucleic acids, RNA and DNA remain intact.

So what the latest studies have inadvertently done is help us realize the infinite richness of this ancient compost. We now know that many, if not all of the health-promoting components found in food and supplements are found intact in this ancient gift to the present – humus. By adding such ancient compost to our soil, Mother Nature gave us the means to return all of the priceless nutrients to our food and water.   This is the basis for mineral assumption and cellular distribution in our vegetables and fruits. By adding chlorine however, we have turned her priceless gifts into a deadly poison. It is similar to King Midas' golden touch, except each element that chlorine touches turns to poison instead of gold.

Consider what happens each time you eat. The fresh plant foods you consume combine with the chlorinated tap water you drink with your meal, or cook your food in, is creating toxins. If you ingest MSG and Aspartame, the toxic load is even greater! Fresh fruits and vegetables, salads, green, black and herb teas, mineral and herbal supplements, MSG, Aspartame, and even certain pharmaceutical drugs, all can turn harmful when combined with chlorine molecules in water. Furthermore, the deadly cancer-causing agents that are produced are extremely toxic in infinitesimal amounts – so small that they are extremely difficult to detect. Similarly, very little chlorine is required to turn your best food into poison. Worse yet, when the concentrations of these health-promoting phytochemicals are high, such as in concentrated health supplements, or even fruits and vegetables coming from highly fertile soils, the deadly combination with chlorination actually intensifies.

This means simply this: if you are taking chlorine into your body through drinking it, bathing or showering in it, or even washing your food in it, you are creating even more poison when you are eating the very best and most organic produce, and taking the best and most nutritious mineral supplements. In addition to not drinking it, cooking with it, or showering or bathing in it, you may want to go through a checklist and look at any other chlorine intake, such as brushing your teeth, rinsing your foods, swimming in a pool, or using a public hot tub or shower where you work out. If you eat out, query your restaurants as whether they filter ALL their water (not just the water they serve!) Many now do. It's not enough to just drink bottled water at a restaurant; what about their soups and their sauces? If they have cooked everything in chlorinated water, it may have already turned many of the vital elements of the food into toxins. On top of this, the restaurant has probably loaded up the food with one or more forms of MSG.

We have erroneously put chlorine into a mental framework of something that is ok to use only in small doses. It absolutely is not! If you give a person small doses of a poison, like arsenic, in time you do indeed murder them.   Once again, Chlorine gas, (often called Mustard Gas) was used extensively in World War I to kill through suffocation.   When we add it to water, the same thing happens – we suffocate nature's most precious gift – the utilization of oxygen molecules.

To be completely sure your water is safe to drink, you need to purchase a home water distiller.   This is the only water that is free of contaminants linked to chlorination.

It is my humble opinion that this message on just how harmful the actions of adding absolute poisons to millions of individuals' culinary water and food supply is of the utmost importance to everyone living in the U.S. and Canada.   It is my prayer that one fine day, the Secret Assassin "toxins" identified in this book will each become exposed as the major cause and contributor to cancer and chronic degenerative disease states that they truly are.   Hopefully people will awaken en masse, and realize that they damage the body's immune and hormonal systems by consuming substances that are designed to alter the food-based proteins, amino acids, and phytochemicals that support those systems.   On that one fine day, the tobacco-industry scandal will simply be dwarfed by comparison! On that one fine day, meaningful reform in our health care system will also of necessity be realized, and human suffering greatly lessened.

[i] **New York Times** newspaper article, January 20, 1979

[ii] The Merck Index, 13th Edition, *Merck Research Laboratories,* 2001 pp 1540-1541

[iii] McKay, F.S. Relation of Mottled Enamel to Caries. J Am Dent Assoc 1928: 15: 1429-37

[iv] Yiamouyiannis, Dr. John. Fluoride: The Aging Factor. Health Action Press 1993 pg 141

[v] Editorial: "Chronic Fluorine Intoxication". Journal of American Medical Association, Volume 31, pp 1360-1363 (1943)

[vi] "Editorial: Effect of Fluorine on Dental Caries.," **Journal of American Dental Association.** Volume 31, (1944)

[vii] Yiamouyiannis, Dr. John. Fluoride: The Aging Factor. Health Action Press 1993, pg 142.

[viii] Griffiths, J. "Fluoride: Commie Plot or Capitalist Ploy" **Covert Action.** Number 24 pp 26-29, 63-66. (1992)

[ix] **J Am Water Works Association,** *1950, 43-6*

[x] **Proceedings of the Fourth Annual Conference of State Dental Directors with the public Health Service and the Children's Bureau, Federal Security Building, Washington, DC, USA 6-8 June 1951**

[xi] "Toxicological Profile for Fluorides, Hydrogen Fluoride, and Fluorine", **U.S. Public Health Service** 1993.

[xii] Groves, Barry **Fluoride: Drinking Ourselves to Death** Gill and MacMillan 2001, pg 227

[xiii] Poklis, A. Mackell MA. "Disposition of fluoride in a fatal case of unsuspected sodium fluoride poisoning." **Forensic Sci Intl.** 1980 Apr.-May 41 55-9

[xiv] WNHO publication Clorination ByProducts and your Health. 1995, pp. 32-26

[xv] Ibid

Chapter 6

Sentencing and Solutions

...perhaps there is a pattern set up in the heavens for one who desires to see it, and having seen it, to find one in himself.
- Plato

Man did not weave the web of life, he is merely a strand in it. Whatever he does to the web, he does to himself.
- Chief Seattle

Knowledge is structured in consciousness. The process of education takes place in the field of consciousness; the prerequisite to complete education is therefore the full development of consciousness – enlightenment. Knowledge is not the basis of enlightenment, enlightenment is the basis of knowledge.
- Maharishi Mahesh Yogi

At the end of most successfully prosecuted trial cases where sickening, oftentimes disgusting and emotionally upsetting testimony is presented, the victims can begin the process of restoring their lives and healing only when and if justice is truly served and a plan of restitution is presented.   Fortunately, in the case against the excitotoxin chemicals Aspartame, MSG, sodium fluoride, chlorine, and their corporate manufacturers, there is indeed a workable plan of restitution.

Fortunately, the human body is a tremendously resilient work of creation. Many times cells, tissues, and even organs such as the brain, damaged by outside invading toxins can repair and regenerate themselves if given the necessary building blocks, and if the offending toxins are removed soon enough.

For instance, consider if you will the amazing miracle of birth. From a single egg, specialized DNA-encoded cells called Stem Cells begin their incredible work. Within just a few weeks, an entirely new human being begins to take shape. Soon, the cells begin to specialize into specific tissues, and then into specific organs such as lungs, kidneys, liver, and the greatest miracle of all – the human brain. In only 9 months, a new human being is ready to become self sufficient, no longer needing a placental cord, with a unique set of fingerprints and individual personality all its own.

The activity of the stem cells in this amazing pageant of life is dependent entirely on the availability and uninterrupted flow of critical building blocks of nutrients, including water, oxygen, and a handful of vital mineral elements such as Calcium, Sodium, Potassium, and Magnesium. If the fetus' mother is deficient in these elements, then birth defects may occur, but not before the physical body of the mother is taxed to the breaking point. For instance, did you know that symptoms of morning sickness in pregnant women (nausea, vomiting, dizziness etc.) are in reality symptoms consistent with chronic dehydration? You see, the stem cells of the fetus draw its nutrients from the mother, especially the specialized water of the amniotic fluid, when the mother is asleep at night and in the deepest level of slumber. Upon awakening the next day, the mother experiences dehydration symptoms, and often does not realize exactly why – only that it is because of her pregnant condition. If she would only drink 20 oz. of ultra-pure water before bedtime, and another 20 oz. in the morning, her "morning sickness" would be much less severe.

Each organ in the developing fetus' body is dependent on specific minerals to achieve optimum growth and complete function. A deficiency in these prime elements often is manifest in the child at some point in their development. This is yet another problem with consuming excitotoxins like MSG and Aspartame when you are pregnant; certain birth defects and developmental abnormalities have been linked to their consumption. Ominously, often times genetic damage to the core DNA does not fully manifest itself until the 2nd or 3rd generation. So, it is very likely still too early to tell the full extent of the damage that excitotoxins may have caused or are still causing the human gene pool.

If you can honestly and objectively count yourself as one of the hundreds of millions of MSG and Aspartame victims who have low energy and are carrying around an extra spare tire (or two) around your midsection because of their toxic effects – a possible answer may be found in the healing and neutralizing effects of a specific combination of water and minerals. After all, isn't this combination what produced your body and your life in the very beginning, as they combined with carbon to form the building blocks of life – amino acids, proteins, vitamins, fats, sugars, complex carbohydrates, etc?

Along with providing the key to growth of the developing fetus in the womb, stem cells also hold the key to the repair and regeneration of damaged neurons and glutamate receptors caused by years of ignorantly consuming chemical excitotoxins. The key to energizing and stimulating the body's stem cells may well be found in the mineral elements provided by Mother Earth. These mineral elements are the very basis of nutrition.

At approximately the same time that monosodium glutamate was poised to invade America, a brilliant medical scientist named Dr. Maynard Murray had made some incredible discoveries. In 1947, Dr. Murray began a 25-year medical career where he specialized in ear, nose and throat treatments. Like most medical professionals with a tender heart and high integrity, Dr. Murray's experiences with his patients aroused in him a deep concern for the quality of life. Even in his era, he could readily see that while Americans were living longer, medical practice statistics revealed that they weren't really living BETTER. Chronic, crippling disease and illness were slowly yet steadily increasing. In his journal he wrote these words: "Americans hold the dubious distinction of being among the sickest of populations in modern society. A nation with a drug industry flourishing as well as ours certainly cannot claim good health!"[i] He knew there had to be a better way, and so he turned his research to the prime elements of nutrition, the minerals on the periodic table of the elements.

Dr. Murray, while still a University student, did some experimentation with cancer cells, inducing the disease in different experimental animals. To his complete surprise, no matter how hard he tried, he could not induce cancer into the body of a toad. The amphibian exhibited a complete natural immunity to all injected cancer cells. He found the same was true in ocean animals and mammals as well. He knew he was onto something big. He spent thousands of his own dollars to travel, study, and dissect sea life from South America to the Pacific Islands.

Dr. Murray sliced open whales, autopsied dolphins and other marine mammals such as seals and sea lions searching for any sign of organic degeneration such as cancer, arthritis, or heart disease. He was amazed that such diseases simply did not exist in the denizens of the sea. He also discovered a species of sea trout that had become land-locked in fresh water. These trout ALL developed liver cancer in 5 years, while he never observed a single cancer in the same species of trout living in sea water – and he autopsied hundreds of specimens. In his journal he penned: "Looking at ocean life, one is immediately impressed that in this 71 percent of earth's surface, there is no cancer, hardening of arteries, or arthritis. Disease resistance in sea plants and animals differs remarkably from land animals. Ocean trout don't develop cancer, while freshwater trout over 5 years have liver cancers. It's difficult to find any land species without cancer. All land animals develop some arteriosclerosis, yet sea animals are never diagnosed with this!"

Murray pondered over what could be the factor that gave this incredible immunity to sea creatures. He found after 30 years of research what exactly that factor was. It was a specific mineral blend. He found that a clean sample of ocean water held EXACTLY the same ratios of primary minerals as healthy human blood. He also found that individuals with different chronic diseases uniformly exhibited imbalanced mineral ratios in their blood.

Here then was the grand key. Trace minerals in correct size and suspension! He discovered much the same truth as his contemporary scientist Dr. Linus Paulings – two time Nobel Prize winner. At the twilight of his remarkably brilliant career, Dr. Paulings declared the following: "You can trace every illness, every disease, and every ailment ultimately to a mineral deficiency."

In analyzing the chemical structure of monosodium glutamate, I discovered that a specific blend of prime minerals might indeed help the brain stem neutralize the toxic effects of this excitotoxin somewhat.   Without going into a science lecture and putting the reader to sleep, suffice it to say that every chemical, every drug, and every prime nutrient that is consumed by the human body on the cellular level produces a specific frequency of vibration that the central nervous system and the brain respond to.   For instance, an aspirin is derived from the bark of a willow tree, and its unique atomic weight and structure provide elements that allow the brain to produce a mild stimulant to the nervous system to relieve the symptoms of pain and swelling.

Mother Nature has a wide variety of remedies in her medicine chest.   But the problem is, unless a pharmaceutical laboratory can artificially manufacture a unique and proprietary chemical chain, and successfully gain patents on it, there is very little profit to be made because every other competitor can produce it as well.   This is the biggest single problem with pharmacopia.

For every synthetic chemical drug produced, there of necessity are numerous and often serious side effects.   This is exactly what happened with American Home Products and Fen-Phen, as outlined in an earlier chapter.   Of course, the executives of AHP had a pretty accurate handle on how popular a prescription weight loss pharmaceutical would be.

However, isn't it much safer, and doesn't it make much more sense to identify and expose one of the prime contributing factors to America's obesity problem?   Why would America's largest pharmaceutical cartel members wish to tip off the American public to what may perhaps be the biggest single threat to their health and well being? The answer is very simple, how much money will they make from a well-balanced, healthy American family that practices sound nutritional principles and is not obese?? They are most definitely hoping that America ignores the warning in this (and other books) about MSG, Aspartame, and other hidden chemical poisons. When you lose your most precious possession, your health, then and only then, do their cash registers begin to ring.

The American health care system is most definitely in need of a major overhaul. At one time in China, a physician was only paid when the family he was treating remained completely healthy. When a family member fell ill, the physician lost his income until health was restored. It seems that our American system is backwards. Our hospitals and medical professionals only get paid when we have a hospital stay, or "come down with" a cold, flu, or other ailment. With the multitude of toxins Americans consume daily, this system ensures a very lucrative income stream, as well as powerful incentives to make "we the people" chronically ill.

If the health of a Nation is in fact tied to the overall wealth of that Nation, then where are the preventative maintenance clinics? Where is the education the public needs to make correct choices? Shouldn't this be one of the top priorities of government, to provide for the general welfare of the populace? Instead, it seems that politicians are a very large part of the problem – receiving fat paychecks from the very same corporations that are anxiously engaged in keeping the people in the dark and completely reliant on (or addicted to) their prescription medications.

Is it really possible that a specific blend of minerals from Mother Earth can actually help the body overcome decades of chemical toxicity? Based on the work of pioneers like Dr. Bernard Jensen, Dr. Gabriel Cousen, Dr. Linus Paulings, and Dr. Maynard Murray, the answer is a resounding YES!!! Just because you haven't heard the story, doesn't mean it is not 100% true. If you question why your doctor hasn't counseled you on this, keep this always in mind – the health care cartel is extremely large, wealthy, and exerts extreme political influence in ALL aspects of American culture and society. The media receives billions in annual revenue from the cartel members to advertise their toxins. Why would they wish to jeopardize their gravy train to promote the facts of science and principles of good health that a simple mineral blend provides? Do you believe that Big Business Buries the Truth?

The truth is, that supplementing your diet with a daily mineral blend that mirrors the ratios of pristine ocean waters with absolutely all industrial, chemical toxins removed, taken sublingually (under the tongue) so that it is 100% absorbed into the blood, will indeed provide the human body with every one of the prime building blocks of good health. Repair and regeneration is the inevitable result.

You must also understand the fact that to be totally effective, a mineral element must be small enough to be absorbed by the cell membrane. This is why consuming fruits and vegetables grown in mineral rich and balanced soil is the best choice. They have absorbed the minerals via osmosis through their root systems. The minerals in fruit and vegetable cells are 1/1000 of a micron in diameter, or in scientific terms, an angstrom in size measurement.

However, as reported to the U.S. Senate in 1936, our croplands have largely become mineral deficient[ii]. So, the next best thing is angstrom-sized mineral suspensions applied under the tongue (sublingually). These products supply the minerals to the blood stream in the correct size, which then allows the internal organs and tissues to utilize the basic mineral in a myriad of biological transmutations. Almost miraculous "healings" can then, and often do occur.

Unlike a synthetic chemical drug that is designed to give immediate relief from symptoms, a program of providing pure nutrition through mineral supplementation often takes weeks and months to produce the desired cessation of symptoms however. We need to understand that whatever health challenge we face, from obesity to heart disease to cancer, it did not happen to us overnight. It took years for the condition to arrive at our doorstep. We cannot logically then expect the condition to disappear overnight with a "magic bullet" pill from our doctor. When we understand that the problem is most likely linked to deficiencies and toxins in the food we consume, then shouldn't we do the best we can to eliminate the problems?

In addition to supplementing minerals in the correct form and drinking purified, distilled water, there are other measures you can take to protect yourself and your loved ones from developing chronic disease symptoms. In recent years, it has become self-evident that many if not all of the neurodegenerative disease states of the central nervous system begin with an impaired energy production system on the cellular level. Dr. Blaylock et. al., have shown in their research, that low ATP (adenison tri-phosphate) levels in the cells makes the cell neurons much more vulnerable to injury by the damaging effects of the toxins exposed in this book. Two natural chemical compounds named L-carnitine and acetyl L-carnitine appear to be able to boost ATP production in the cells, thus giving the body a greater margin of protection from the toxic barrage. One of the very best liquid supplements to provide L-carnitine, as well as a wonderful stand-alone liquid mineral product is distributed by Sageant Company, 1-888-777-4612.

As is typically the case, nature often provides antidotes for all toxins, very often from the same forest glen that produces the poison. From the shores of postwar Japan, a possible antidote to MSG toxicity created by Japan's Ajinomoto appears very promising.

In 1951, postwar Japan was facing a serious problem, a food shortage. The wealthy industrial corporate citizens such as Ajinomoto had little concern, but the average Japanese family was in dire straits. Dr. Hiroshi Tamiya discovered a technology to successfully grow, harvest, and process a 2.5 billion year old alga named Chlorella.

Dr. Tamiya was well aware of the history of Chlorella. He knew that it had been on the earth since the Precambrian period, and had survived countless changes in the earth's climate. He knew also that human eyes under a microscope first identified chlorella cells in the 1890's. Dr. Tamiya had been working with a joint chlorella research program with scientists in Germany since the late 1920's. They had discovered that chlorella consisted of 60% protein, and yet nothing they had ever witnessed grew and multiplied so rapidly. They rightfully concluded that chlorella could well be the food of the future, and that it could be successfully grown on a commercial scale. Chlorella was the first form of life to develop a true cellular nucleus. It is a powerful producer of chlorophyll, and reproduces itself by cell division at the astounding rate of 4 new cells every 17-24 hours.

Dr. Tamiya did not see his dream of chlorella as a source of the world's food come to pass. His team had uncovered a problem. Chlorella's tough cell wall was largely non-digestible, and passed unscathed though the human digestion tract. Japanese ingenuity solved the problem of digestibility in 1975, when a patented procedure was developed that naturally breaks down the chlorella cell walls and yields a digestibility rate of over 80%. In the 80's, Japanese scientists turned their attention to the possibilities of chlorella as a promoter of good health. Upon analysis, it was found that chlorella contains an astonishingly wide variety of natural vitamins and minerals, along with an impressive assortment of essential amino acids. Additionally, it has many other unknown factors such as Chlorella Growth Factor (CGF) that scientists are only now beginning to fully understand. These "unknown growth factors" have been shown to be the reason chlorella greatly increases the absorption and bio-availability of minerals in human cells. It also promotes the healing of damaged neurons. [iii]

Experiments with microorganisms, animals and children have shown that chlorella promotes faster than normal growth without adverse side effects. In adults, it appears to enhance RNA/DNA functions responsible for the production of proteins, enzymes and ATP energy at the cellular level. It has been shown to be able to stimulate tissue repair and protects the cells against excitotoxin damage.[iv]

Another very vital nutritional supplement that I would highly recommend is the hormone called melatonin. Produced naturally in the pineal gland of the human brain, melatonin production is highest in pre-pubescent children, and is commonly called the "sleep hormone". After puberty, melatonin production gradually decreases as the body ages. Melatonin levels also have been shown to decrease under periods of stress. This is why people under high stress often have problems sleeping through the night, and if the stress level is not reduced disease states often form. The primary reason for this is because stress causes melatonin levels to decrease. Melatonin is produced by the pineal gland from protein molecules. Be sure to consume ONLY ALL-NATURAL, NON-SYNTHETIC, NON-ANIMAL melatonin however. There are numerous companies that produce melatonin – and the vast majority are synthetic chemicals, much like MSG and Aspartame. The pure, natural melatonin from vegetable protein in liquid, sublingually applied form, blended with minerals can be purchased from Vance's Foods, Inc., 1-800-822-6980.

I would submit that the height of lunacy is expecting a different end result without substantially changing the pattern and design of our actions. As Einstein said, doing the same thing over and over again and expecting different results is the definition of stupidity. Fortunately, there are indeed companies seeking solutions to these very grave problems. For a complete list of just a few companies that I highly recommend, turn to the addendum located in the back of this book.

---

[i] Murray, Dr. Maynard; Sea Energy Agriculture

[ii] Senate Document No. 264, Year – 1936. 74th Congress, 2nd Session. (See Addendum for verbatim, unabridged extracts.)

[iii] Hasegawa T, Kimura Y, et al."Effect of hot water extract of Chlorella vulagaris on cytokine expression patterns in mice with murine acquired immunodeficiency syndrome after infection with Listeria monocytogenes." **Immunopharmacology, 1997 Jan;** 35(3):273-82

[iv] Tanaka K; Koga T; Konishi F, "Augmentation of host defense by a unicellular green alga, Chlorella vulgaris" **Infectious Immunology 1986 Aug;**53(2):267-71

NOTES

Chapter 7

A New Life – Out on Parole

Words ought to be a little wild, for they are the assaults of thoughts on the
unthinking.

- John Maynard Keynes

To put the world in order, we must first put the nation in order; to put the nation in
order, we must put the family in order; to put the family in order, we must cultivate
our personal life; and to cultivate our personal life, we must first set our hearts right.
- Confucius

Like millions of other Americans in the same age group, James, 46, was noticeably slowing down. He just couldn't seem to do the things he enjoyed doing, even a decade ago. He worked his whole life in the construction trade, and it was getting more and more difficult to put in a full day of work. It seemed that his joints and muscles ached continuously. He had slowly been gaining weight, and that large belly of his still seemed to increase no matter what diet he tried. He would lose 10 pounds or so, but then would gain 15 more in short order a month or so later. His doctor informed him when he went in last winter for help getting over the flu that his cholesterol was in the danger zone, and he gave him a prescription to lower it. The trouble is, while he couldn't prove it, he felt that the prescription made him irritable and unable to sleep well. His wife told him that even if that were true, it was a small price to pay for lowering his risk for heart attack or stroke.

Then a friend invited him to go to a meeting where a gentleman was lecturing on nutrition. This man talked about something called exitotoxins and taught James about the hidden chemicals in his food. James at first was skeptical. Next, he reviewed the many studies on the subject. Could losing weight, regaining his youthful energy and vitality, getting off prescription drugs, and enjoying life to the fullest once again really be as easy as eliminating these toxic chemicals and taking a simple mineral supplement? James decided to give it a try, and made the commitment to change his life for at least the next 6 months.

James and his wife Jennifer soon realized however, that committing to the program was not as easy as it sounded. They began to read labels, and to their chagrin, found that virtually all of their favorite dishes were loaded with 2, 3 or even more MSG-laden ingredients. They hadn't realized that they needed to eliminate virtually all processed and packaged foods. However, they had made the commitment, and still were determined to make the changes.

The first two weeks were not easy; in fact they were very difficult. Both James and Jennifer noticed a dull, throbbing headache especially in the morning. Their aches, pains, and joint stiffness were markedly worse. They noticed they were very short tempered and irritable. But that is exactly what that crazy nutritionist told them would happen. He had told them that they would experience withdrawal/detoxification symptoms – just as they would experience from giving up any other chemical drug that they had become addicted to over time. Often they were tempted to grab a bucket of chicken or a handful of potato chips, however, they successfully fought the urges.

Almost magically, on the 22nd day of their new diet, things started to change. They both noticed a pronounced new sense of well-being. They had a marked increase in energy levels. Their sleep was deeper and much more restful. At the end of their respective workdays, they even had enough energy to take long walks around their neighborhood together. And more incredibly, they fully enjoyed the experience. The air smelled fresher, and they even looked forward to family outings and campouts. Their energy levels had markedly increased. Hikes and other activities became enjoyable again.

Before they knew it, 6 months had passed. But James and Jennifer realized they had another problem. Their clothes no longer fit them. They had each lost over 30 pounds and many inches from their waistlines. Their friends and neighbors noticed the difference as well. They looked great. They wondered what health club they had joined and exactly what they were doing. Of course, James and Jennifer are all too eager to share the information that changed their lives so much.

If you want to experience the same excitement and zest of life and living that a young child possesses, then follow the steps outlined in this book. It is in fact based on sound science and basic principles. You do not need to follow a rigid diet regimen per se. You need to continue to eat reasonable amounts of pure meats, fruits, nuts, and vegetables and eliminate MSG laden foods. It is amazing and absolutely exciting.

The friend that shared this book with you can also share with you the products that have been specially designed to help you and your loved ones eliminate and lessen the effects of excitotoxins on your life. They can also give you the support you need to continue to eliminate these poisons from your diet.   Preparing new and wholesome food dishes does not need to be a troublesome task – with the help of a group of like-minded individuals sharing recipes and tips, your new life can be a lot of fun.

Remember that a new life complete with a new waistline and wardrobe is not a destination, but rather an ongoing journey. Rest assured, the rewards are well worth the effort. It is time to begin NOW. There is no reason to delay. Make the conscious decision to change and stick with it. You will be glad you did.

By reading this book, you have unmasked the Ninja, the Secret Assassins that are attacking your health and well-being. When a Ninja loses his ability to move covertly, his power is largely negated, as is his ability to destroy.

A Ninja is also defined as a paid assassin. In the Oriental culture, Ninjas are not inexpensive to employ. They are highly skilled in their covert death trade. More often than not, their victim dies silently without a clue or a hint of the attack. For this reason, Ninjas are very selective as to who employs them. There is often a geo-political motive behind their assault. They wish to further social upheaval and foment changes.

America is the greatest nation in modern history. America became great, not only because of our goodness, justice and mercy, but primarily because we the people have loved freedom and have been willing to fight and die to protect it.   The silent Secret Assassins, the Ninjas of Taste outlined in the pages of this book, have been attacking this nation systematically since WW II. Our freedoms are being eroded like never before. Can we remain a truly free and independent nation if the vast majority of us are obese diabetics with dysfunctional brains?   What kind of world will we bequeath to our posterity, our children and grandchildren?   What genetic deformities will they experience in succeeding generations thanks to "recombinant DNA" technologies? More importantly, will we continue to allow Big Business to Bury the Truth?

Congratulations, if you say the answer is NO!

THE NEW BEGINNING

(Not really The End!)

ADDENDUM

Verbatim Unabridged Extracts from the 74th Congress, 2nd Session

"Our physical well being is more directly dependent upon the minerals we take into our systems than upon calories or vitamins, or upon the precise proportions of starch, protein or carbohydrates we consume."

"Do you know that most of us today are suffering from certain dangerous diet deficiencies which cannot be remedied until depleted soils from which our food come are brought into proper mineral balance?"

"The alarming fact is that foods (fruits, vegetables, and grains) now being raised on millions or acres of land that no longer contains enough of certain minerals are starving us – no matter how much of then we eat. No man of today, can eat enough fruits and vegetables to supply his system with the minerals he requires for perfect health because his stomach isn't big enough to hold them."

"The truth is that our foods vary enormously in value, and some of them aren't worth eating as food. Again, our physical well-being is more directly dependent upon the minerals we take into our systems than upon calories or vitamins or upon the precise proportions of starch, protein or carbohydrates we consume."

"This talk about minerals is novel and quite startling. In fact, a realization of the importance of minerals in food is so new that the textbooks on nutritional dietetics contain very little about it. Nevertheless, it is something that concerns all of us, and the further we delve into it the more startling it becomes."

"You'd think, wouldn't you, that a carrot is a carrot – that one is about as good as another as far as nourishment is concerned? But it isn't; one carrot , may look and taste like another and yet be lacking in the particular mineral element which our system requires and which carrots are supposed to contain."

"Laboratory tests prove that the fruits, the vegetables, the grains, the eggs, and even the milk and the meats of today are not what they were a few generations ago (which doubtless explains why our forefathers thrived on a selection of foods that would starve us!)"

" No man today can eat enough fruits and vegetables to supply his stomach with the mineral salts he requires for perfect health, because his stomach isn't big enough to hold them! And we are turning into big stomachs!"

" No longer does a balanced and fully nourishing diet consists of merely so many calories or certain vitamins or fixed proportions of starches, proteins and carbohydrates. We know that our diets must contain in addition something like a score of minerals salts."

" It is bad news to learn from our leading authorities that 99% of the American people are deficient in these minerals, and that a marked deficiency in any one of the more important minerals actually results in disease. Any upset of the balance, any considerable lack of one or another element, however microscopic the body requirement may be, and we sicken, suffer, and shorten our lives."

" We know that vitamins are complex chemical substances, which are indispensable to nutrition, and that each of them is of importance for normal function of some special structure in the body. Disorder and disease result from any vitamin deficiency. It is not commonly realized, however, that vitamins control the body's appropriation of minerals, and in the absence of minerals they have no function to perform. Lacking vitamins, the system can make some use of minerals, but lacking minerals, vitamins are USELESS!"

" This discovery is one of the latest and most important contributions of science to the problem of human health."

Outlets for Mineral and Nutritional Products

David Wolfe – www.rawfood.com

San Diego, CA

DAVID HAS THE LOWEST PRICES ON RAW & LIVING FOOD PRODUCTS ANYWHERE, GUARANTEED!!!
For phone orders, call toll free 1-800-205-2350 or (619) 596-7979

Southern Herb Company, LLC

http://www.southernherb.com/catalog/index.php

Sageant Company, LLC

Home Office: Bozeman, MT

www.sageant.com

Tel: 1-888-777-4612

Vance's Incorporated

Home Office: Soldotna, AK

www.vances.com

Tel: 1-800-822-6980

Mother Earth Minerals, Inc.

Ogden, Utah

www.motherearthmineralsinc.com

Tel: 1-866-989-9876

Cocoon Nutrition

274 E Hamilton Avenue, Ste. G

Campbell, CA 95008

www.cocoonnutrition.org

Tel: 888-988-3325

IN THE SENATE OF THE UNITED STATES
    AUGUST 1 (LEGISLATIVE DAY, JULY 16), 1985
Mr. Metzenbaum introduced the following bill; which was read twice and
referred to the Committee on Labor and Human Resources

_____

A BILL

To provide the public with information concerning the use of products
containing aspartame, to provide for the conduct of studies to
determine the health effects of using products containing aspartame,
and for other purposes.

Be it enacted by the Senate and House of Representatives of the United
States of America in Congress assembled, that this Act may be cited as
the "Aspartame Safety Act of 1985"

    LABELING REQUIREMENTS

    SEC. 2. (a) Section 403 of the Federal Food, Drug, and Cosmetic
Act is amended by adding at the end thereof the following new
paragraph:
    "(q)(1) If it contains aspartame, unless its label and labeling--

    "(A) specify the total number of milligrams of aspartame
contained in each serving;
    "(B) specify the allowable daily intake of aspartame (in
milligrams) for each kilogram of human body weight, as established by
the Secretary; and
    "C) bear the following statement: "THIS PRODUCT CONTAINS
ASPARTAME, WHICH IS NOT INTENDED FOR USE IN INFANT FEEDING'".
    "(2) The Secretary shall be regulation require that the
information required by subparagraph (1)(B) to be specified on the
label and labeling of any food containing aspartame be included on such
label and labeling in a manner which is the most useful to individuals
who consume such food.
    "(3)   The statement required by subparagraph (1)(C) shall be
located in a conspicuous place on the label and labeling of each food
containing aspartame as proximate as possible to the name of such food
and shall appear in conspicuous and legible type in contrast by
typography, layout, and color with other printed matter on such label
and labeling.".
    (b)(1) Section 502 of such Act is amended by adding at the end
thereof the following new paragraph:
    "(u)(1) If it is a drug containing aspartame, unless--
        "(A) its label and labeling--
            "(i) specify the total number of milligrams of
aspartame contained in each dosage;
            "(ii) specify the allowable daily intake of aspartame
(in milligrams) for each kilogram of human body weight, as established
by the Secretary; and
            "(iii) bear the following statements:
    'THIS PRODUCT CONTAINS ASPARTAME, AND IS NOT INTENDED FOR USE BY
INFANTS', PHENYLKETONURICS: CONTAINS PHENYLALANINE'; and
            "(B) the manufacturer, packer, or distributor (including all
retail establishments) thereof includes in all advertisements and other

printed and descriptive matter issued or caused to be issued by the
manufacturer, packer, or distributor with respect to such drug the
information described in clauses (A)(i) and (A)(ii) and the statements
specified in clause (A)(iii).".

"(2) The Secretary shall by regulation require that the
information required by subparagraph (1)(A)(ii) to be specified on the
label and labeling of drugs containing aspartame be included on such
label and labeling in a manner which is the most useful to individuals
who consume such drugs.

"(3) The statements required by subparagraph (1)(A)(iii) shall be
located in a conspicuous place on the label and labeling of each drug
containing aspartame as proximate as possible to the name of such drug
and shall appear in conspicuous and legible type in contrast by
typography, layout, and color with other printed matter on such label
and labeling.".

(2) The first sentence of section 503(b)(2) of such Act is
amended by striking out "and (1)," and inserting in lieu therefore of
"(1), and(u)(1)(B),".

MORATORIUM

SEC. 3.   During the period beginning on the date of enactment of
this Act and ending--
        (1) on the date which is one year after the date of enactment
of this Act, or
        (2) the date on which all studied required under section 4 are
completed, whichever is earlier, the Secretary of Health and Human
Services (hereinafter referred to as the "Secretary") shall not approve
or permit any use of aspartame in any food or drug if such use was not
approved or permitted on the date of enactment of this Act.

RESEARCH

SEC. 4 (a) The Secretary, through the Director of the National
Institutes of Health, shall request proposals for, and make grants and
enter into contracts for the conduct of, clinical studies on aspartame,
including studies concerning--
        (1) the effect of the consumption of aspartame on brain chemistry;
        (2) the health effects of the consumption of aspartame on pregnant
women and fetuses;
        (3) behavioral and neurological effects experienced by individuals
who have consumed aspartame, especially by children who have consumed
aspartame;
        (4) the interaction of aspartame with drugs, including monoamine
oxidase inhibitors, alpha-methyl-dopa, and L-dihydroxphenylalanine; and
        (5) the effect of the consumption of aspartame in increasing the
probability of seizures.
    (b) In making grants and entering into contracts under subsection
(a), the Secretary shall provide for the completion of the studies
required under such subsection with one year after the date of
enactment of this Act.
    (c) To carry out this section, there are authorized to be
appropriated such sums as may be necessary.
    (d) The authority of the Secretary to enter into contracts under this
section shall be to such extend or in such amounts as are provided in
appropriation Acts.

174

CLINICAL ADVERSE REACTION COMMITTEE ON ASPARTAME

SEC. 5. (a) The Secretary, through the Commissioner of the Food and Drug Administration, shall establish a Clinical Adverse Reaction Committee on Aspartame. The Committee shall collect reports of individual reactions the consumption of foods containing aspartame, including reports of reactions from individuals taking various medications, and shall evaluate and prepare appropriate responses to such reports.

(b) The Secretary shall announce the establishment of the Committee under subsection (a) through the mailing of written notices to physicians and other health care providers and through advertisements in medical journals and in publications read by the general public. Such advertisements shall include the telephone number of the service established pursuant to subsection (c).

(c) The Secretary shall establish a telephone service for the reporting by individuals of reactions to the consumption of products containing aspartame. Calls on such telephone service shall be without charge to the caller.

****

Note 1: It is my understanding that this bill was bottled up in committee and essentially killed by Senator Orrin Hatch.

Note 2: It is also my understanding that by virtue of the FDA classification of this substance, NO reports of adverse reactions were required or wanted.

Letter from Senator Howard Metzenbaum on United States Senate Stationery (Committee on the Budget) dated February 3, 1986 to Orrin Hatch who was the Chairman of the Labor and Human Resources Committee, Metzenbaum was a member of this committee, along with Ted Kennedy, Strom Thurmond, Lowell Weicker, Christopher Dodd, Dan Quale, John Kerry and others.

Dear Orrin;

NutraSweet, manufactured by the G.D. Searle Company, is currently being consumed in ever-increasing amounts by over 100 million Americans. Last year, Americans consumed over 20 billion cans of diet soft drinks, the vast majority of which were sweetened with 100 percent NutraSweet. The average consumer assumes that all safety questions surrounding this sweetener had been resolved long before it found its way onto every grocery shelf in America.

A recent investigation under taken by my office raises serious questions as to whether this is, in fact, the case. These questions can only be resolved by Congressional hearings, with full subpoena power, being undertaken by the Senate Judiciary and labor Committees.

In addition, the facts uncovered by my investigation coupled with concerns expressed in the scientific community regarding the safety of this food additive, compel the immediate initiation of new, truly independent safety tests on NutraSweet.

My concern focuses on the failure of the U.S. Attorney's Office in Chicago to undertake a grand jury investigation of NutraSweet which was requested by the Food and Drug Administration. The investigation was to focus on possible criminal charges against officials in the G. D. Searle Company "for concealing material facts and making false statements" in reports of safety tests on NutraSweet and the drug, Aldactone. (Doc#1)

NutraSweet was first approved by the FDA in 1974. However, concerns about the credibility of Searle's tests led the Investigation Task Force to stay that approval in December, 1975. In 1976, an FDA investigation Task Force published a report on the testing practices at G.D. Searle Company and concluded: "At the heart of FDA's regulatory process is its ability to rely upon the integrity of the basic safety data submitted by sponsors of regulated products. Our investigation clearly demonstrated that, in the G.D. Searle Company, we have no basis for such reliance now." (Doc#2)

One of the recommendations of the FDA's 1976 Task Force Report was that the agency should ask the U.S. Attorney in the Northern District of Illinois to institute grand jury proceedings against G.D. Searle.

It is a matter of public record that in January, 1977, the FDA formally requested that the U.S. Attorney conduct a grand jury investigation of tests on two Searle products; NutraSweet and Aldactone, a drug to treat hypertension. It is also known that the U.S. Attorney declined to prosecute in December, 1978. What has not been publicly known until now is what happened in between.

Following an investigation by my office, the following facts have been established.

   The first U.S. Attorney in charge of the case Samuel Skinner did not convene a grand jury. A year after he was initially informed of FDA's interest in prosecuting Searle, and two months after he received the agency's formal request for grand jury action, he "recused" himself from the case, citing preliminary employment discussions with the law firm of Sidley and Austin, the firm which was then defending Searle in the investigation. He asked his subordinates to keep his discussions confidential "to avoid any undue embarrassment upon the firm of Sidley and Austin." (emphasis supplied).Doc#10). Mr. Skinner joined Sidley and Austin four months later.

Sidley and Austin requested a meeting with Mr. Skinner "prior to the submission to the grand jury of any matters relating to this company." (Doc#6) When the meeting was held, Mr. Newton Minow attended (Doc.#7) Mr. Minow is the partner at Sidley and Austin who offered Mr. Skinner his job with the firm (Doc#8). The meeting was held a month prior to Mr. Skinner "recusing" himself from the case.

In his recusal letter, Mr. Skinner stated his understanding that the decision as to whether or not a grand jury investigation should be conducted would await the arrival of a new U.S. Attorney. (A period which lasted four months). (Doc.#11).

However, no grand jury action was taken before the appointment of a new U.S. Attorney.

This four month delay in the grand jury investigation took place at a time when nearly four and a -half years of a five year statute of limitations on the NutraSweet tests cited by the FDA had already expired.

Shortly after the appointment of the new U.S. Attorney, Mr. Thomas Sullivan, the FDA wrote to Justice noting the delays which had occurred in the case and urged the U. S. Attorney, to " proceed expeditiously." The FDA also cited additional problems they had discovered with a key NutraSweet safety test and noted "further criminal culpability-- the failure to report these problems to the FDA-- may also be revealed which could require submission to the grand jury." (Doc#16).

The Justice Department also wrote to Mr. Sullivan a month after he assumed office complaining about the amount of time which had transpired on the case. Letter states Justice knows of no reason why "grand jury should not at least investigate." (Doc#17).

By the time any case agianst Searle was presented to the grand jury, NutraSweet was dropped from the investigation. This means the issue of whether tests on NutraSweet were fraudulent, which was raised by the 1976 task Force Report, was never put to the grand jury.

We have been informed by Justice there is no record of the U.S. Attorney writing to the FDA to inform the agency that the investigation would proceed on Aldactone alone.

According to a Justice Department memo, (Doc#21), Mr. William Conlon, the Senior Assistant U.S. Attorney assigned to the Searle case "reduced or ended" his involvement in the investigation eighteen months after first being assigned to the case. One year later he accepted a position with Sidley and Austin, the firm which represented Searle in the investigation. (DOC#28).

Key seizure test on NutraSweet was never investigated by grand jury. During a Searle sponsored monkey test, all the animals receiving medium or high dosages of NutraSweet experienced Grand mal Seizures (Doc#28). Searle never performed autopsies. The FDA said Searle made at least four false statements and entries in the report of the study. (Doc#1). Though the FDA later claimed it did not rely on the study to prove safety, the seizures were never explained. Failure to account for these seizures is of particular significance given current concerns expressed in the scientific community on precisely this issue. In the November 9, 1985, edition of Lancet , a recognized authority on brain chemistry, Dr. Richard Wurtman, cited case studies which suggest an association between NutraSweet and Grand Mal seizures. (Doc#29).

Test on key breakdown component of NutraSweet, DKP, was never investigated by grand jury. In July, 1977, the FDA wrote to Justice telling them that FDA inspectors were reviewing a key test on DKP, which raise issues that "could require submission to the grand jury." The U.S. Attorney never submitted the test to the grand jury." In the conducting of the study tissue masses were not reported and uterine polyps were discovered. (Doc#30)

It is a matter of public record that back in 1970, the G.D. Searle Company drew up a "strategy memo" on how to get NutraSweet approved by the FDA. In the memo, they committed themselves to obtaining a favorable review of NutraSweet by seeking to develop within FDA personnel a "subconscious spirit of participation" in the Searle studies. The memo emphasized the importance of getting the FDA in the "habit of saying yes", by first submitting to the FDA those safety issues involving little or no breakdown of NutraSweet into DKP. (Doc#31).

In-House FDA memos showing credibility of key tumor tests were questioned by FDA scientists prior to Commissioner Hayes' approval of NutraSweet. The problems with the credibility of Searle's tests on NutraSweet continued right up to the time FDA Commissioner Hayes overruled a public board of inquiry and approved the food additive in 1981.

Two months prior to approval, the Commissioner was advised by three of his own scientists that three key tumor tests, including the test on DKP, were questionable and that safety had not been proven.   (Doc#26)

I am attaching to this letter a time-line which will highlight the sequence of these events. I am also including an extensive list of documents relating to the grand jury investigation. These documents raise the question as to whether the investigation of the G.D. Searle Company and in particular, the food additive, NutraSweet, was properly conducted.

We will not be able to answer that question without Congressional hearings, with full subpoena power.

As I mentioned earlier, NutraSweet is a product currently being used by 100 million Americans. The fact that a grand jury never investigated charges that Searle concealed "material facts" and made "false statements" (Doc#1) on NutraSweet tests is a matter of serious concern. One can only speculate on what a grand jury with full investigative powers would have uncovered and how that information in turn would have affected the credibility of those tests in the approval process.

There are also the concerns being voiced by scientists over whether key questions of safety have been adequately resolved.

I am including a brief synopsis of recent scientific work raising questions about NutraSweet.

In conclusion, we have a grand jury which never investigated whether criminal fraud was committed on NutraSweet tests, coupled with continuing concerns being expressed in the scientific community regarding this food additive's safety.

I urge you, Orrin, to hold oversight hearings on the health concerns

which have been raised about NutraSweet. It is the only way we can hope
to dispel the cloud hanging over the food additive presently being
consumed in massive quantities by the American people.

Very sincerely yours,

Howard M. Metzenbaum
United States Senator

Letter from Senator Howard Metzenbaum of the Senate Committe on Labor
and Human Resources to Senator Orrin Hatch, the Chairman of the Senate
Committee on Labor and Human Resources

February 25, 1986

Dear Orrin:

I am at a loss to comprehend the thrust of your recent letters on my
request for hearings on the safety concerns raised in the scientific
community regarding NutraSweet.

When I sent you a 110-page report on February 6 on the failure of the
U.S. Attorney to hold a grand jury investigation, you replied the same
day that there were no health issues raised. You then asked that I
share with you all information raising safety issues. Orrin, the report
I sent you included a summary of current health concerns raised by nine
different scientists. My report contained all the relevant references
to medical journals and other citations.

Now you have sent me another letter, dated February 18, in which you
again request evidence.

As you know, I met last Thursday with Dr. Roger Coulombe of Utah State
University. You also had a conversation with Dr. Coulombe, as did your
staff.

Dr. Coulombe has informed both of us that his study of NutraSweet's
effects on brain chemistry contains new and significant data.

All of the 12 mice tested showed brain chemistry changes after
ingesting NutraSweet.

Four other mice received no NutraSweet and showed no brain chemistry
changes. Dr. Coulombe also informed us that the issues raised in his
study were not tested prior to NutraSweet's approval. So, the FDA
never reviewed this research prior to approving NutraSweet.

It is critical to note that some of the lab animals which had reactions
to NutraSweet were fed doses at levels currently being consumed by
humans.

As you know, there have been many reports of seizures, headaches, mood
alterations, etc., associated with NutraSweet. Dr. Coulombe's study,
which has been accepted for publication in Toxicology and Applied
Pharmacology, states:

It is therefore possible that Aspartame may produce
neurobiochemical and behavioral effects in humans, particularly in
children and susceptible individuals. Based on the foregoing, there is
a need for additional research on the safety of this food additive.
Orrin, you have asked for new and significant scientific evidence about
NutraSweet. Now you have it. Dr. Coulombe's research as well as the
other research cited in my report raises new health concerns which have
not been resolved.

We need to hold hearings on NutraSweet-- which is being used by over
100 million Americans. With an issue that is critical to the health of
half the American population, how can you in good conscience say "no?"
We cannot rely upon the tests sponsored by the manufacturer of
NutraSweet, G. D. Searle, and ignore the concerns being raise by
independent studies.

We don't need the company which is making hundreds of millions of
dollars on this product telling us it's "safe," particularly when the
credibility of that Company's testing on NutraSweet has been severely
undermined. You know that the FDA recommended a criminal investigation
of possible fraud in NutraSweet tests. The FDA has never before or
since made such an investigation.

Although NutraSweet was later approved, credible scientific concerns
continue to be raised.

The Director of Clinical Research at M.I.T., Dr. Richard Wurtman, has
recently published a letter in Lancet citing case reports suggesting a
possible association between Aspartame and seizures. According to Dr.
Wurtman, the reports are compatible with evidence that high Aspartame
doses may produce neurochemical changes that, in laboratory animals,
are associated with depressed seizure thresholds.

Dr. William Pardridge, U.C.L.A. School of Medicine, has also cited a
possible link between one of Aspartame's principal components,
phenylalanine, and the lowering lowering of seizure thresholds in
individual\individuals. He has also questioned the possible affects of
NutraSweet on fetal development.

In July, 1985, Dr. Michael Mahalik of the Philadelphia College of
Osteopathic Medicine, and Dr. Ronald Gautieri of Temple University
School of Pharmacy, published a study on the potential of Aspartame to
produce brain dysfunction in mouse neonates whose mothers were exposed
to Aspartame in late gestation. They concluded that the possibility of
brain dysfunction appears to be a viable sequela to excessive Aspartame
exposure.

In June of last year, Dr. Adrian Gross, a former FDA Toxicologist,
and member of the FDA Investigative Task Force which reviewed the
Aspartame studies, sent me a letter stating that depute their serious
shortcomings, at least those studies established beyond a reasonable
doubt that Aspartame is capable of inducing brain tumors in
experimental
animals.

In February, 1985, letters were published in the Annals of Internal

Medicine and the American Journal of Psychiatry, linking Aspartame to skin lesions and to severe headaches caused by chemical interactions with an anti-depressant drug, an M.A.O. inhibitor.

In December, 1984, Dr. John Olney of Washington University published a study on excitotoxic amino acids including Aspartate, one of Aspartame's two constituent amino acids. He concludes that excitotoxins pose a significant hazard to the developing nervous systems of young children.

Dr. Louis Elsas, at Emory University, has raised concerns about Aspartame's other constituent amino acid, phenylalanine. He has stated that if the mother's blood phenylalanine is raise to high concentrations in pregnancy, her child's brain development can be damaged. According to Dr. Elsas, it has not been determined how high the blood phenylalanine must be elevated to produce any of these effects. However, he believes that it has not been proven that all people can take as much Aspartame without fear of ill effects as they desire.

Appearing on the news program Nightline in May of last year, Dr. Elsas warned of a whitewashed scientific review, most of which has been supported by the industry itself, which has obvious conflict of interest.

All of these safety concerns have been raised after NutraSweet was approved for use in over 90 products. The FDA is currently considering petitions which would explain even further the dramatic increase in NutraSweet consumption. My staff has provided you with the references for all of the scientific concerns raised above. I strongly urge you to reconsider your decision and to convene oversight hearings in the Labor and Human Resources Committee as soon as possible to consider these issues.

By ignoring the safety concerns which have been raised, we are potentially jeopardizing the health and safety of over 100 million Americans who are ingesting NutraSweet in everything from soft drinks to pudding to children's cold remedies.

Very Sincerely Yours,

Howard M. Metzenbaum
United Stated Senator

About the Authors

A. True Ott, PhD

Dr. Ott received his Bachelors of Arts degree from Southern Utah University in Cedar City, Utah in 1982, and went on to receive his Doctor of Philosophy in the field of Nutrition through the American College in Washington DC in 1994. Dr. Ott's dissertation followed the groundbreaking work of Linus Pauling, and asserted via independent research that each mineral on the periodic table of the elements, in its pure hexagonal crystalline form, resonates a specific hertz resonant frequency based on its atomic weight and unique electron configuration. Dr. Ott then measured and graphed the individual resonant frequencies inherent in vitamin and enzyme structures, and independently verified that 23 minerals are the base raw materiele of nutrition and are vitally important in keeping the human cells in a state of balance or homeostatic health.

Dr. Ott's research also verified the importance of free electrons in nutritional supplements, including drinking water and oxygen molecules. He developed a patent-pending drinking water product that attaches free electrons to the Hydrogen and Oxygen molecules in ultra-pure, medicinal grade water - making it negatively charged (extra 'free electrons') and then introduced it to individuals suffering from chronic conditions such as diabetes, arthritis, heart disease, etc. Amazingly, the free electrons in Dr. Ott's water product began to reduce the symptoms associated with chronic disease in a very powerful way. As Dr. Ott declared in a recent symposium: "Society has unfortunately taken Water for granted. When I share my research on water and minerals with others in the allopathic medical community, the typical response is mocking derision. Too often health care professionals forget that the human body is composed of 70% water and 30% minerals - and pure water combined with pure minerals comprise Mother Earth's medicine chest for all mammalian life forms! It is not rocket science, only common sense!"

The author and publisher of dozens of articles and three books on nutrition, Dr. Ott is continually searching for natural solutions and answers to the nation's chronic health problems, and believes that education is the first step.

Linda Kozel Hegstand, MD, PhD

Education

1982 – 1986	**M.D.**, University of Wisconsin Medical School, Madison, WI
1969 – 1973	**Ph.D.**, University of Wisconsin – Madison (Biochemistry)
1965 – 1969	**B.A.**, Hope College, Holland, MI, (Chem.), Magna Cum Laude
1962 – 1965	East Rockford Senior High School, Rockford, IL, Salutatorian

Postgraduate Training

1993 – 1994	**Fellow, Surgical Pathology and Hematopathology**, Danbury Hospital, Yale – affiliated, Danbury CT
1986 – 1990	**Internship and Residency in Anatomic and Clinical Pathology**, University of Wisconsin Medical School, Madison, WI
1977 – 1978	**Fellow, Clinical Pharmacology**, University of Colorado Medical School, Denver, CO
1973 – 1977	**Fellow, Pharmacology**, Yale University School of Medicine in the Laboratory of Dr. Paul Greengard, New Haven, CT, Nobel Laureate

Clinical Consultant

1994 – 1999	**Beckman Coulter**: for Access Immunoassay analyzer with emphasis on Cardiac Markers
1994 – 1999	**Dade Behring**: for Sysmex Coagulation analyzers with emphasis on monitoring of anticoagulation

Academic Honors

Society for Pediatric Pathologists Award for most outstanding poster, 1989
Inbusch Award for Outstanding Research (UW-Madison), 1986
Who's Who in International Medicine
Who's Who in the Midwest
Mortar Board (Women's National Honorary Society)
Woodrow Wilson Fellowship (Honorable Mention)
American Institute of Chemists' Award (Michigan)
Faculty Honors (Hope College)
Hope College Honor Scholarship
Outstanding Sophomore Chemistry Award

Professional Memberships

American Academy of Environmental Medicine
American Nutraceutical Association
Michigan State Medical Society
Kent County Medical Society

Teaching Responsibilities

1994 – 1999	Education both written and oral regarding laboratory medicine to Attending Physicians, Resident Physicians, Medical Technologists, Phlebotomists, and Nursing Staff at Spectrum Health and affiliates
1994 – 1997	GRAMEC Pathology Council, Assistant Residency Director
1988 – 1990	Laboratory Instructor in General Pathology for medical students, University of Wisconsin Medical School, Madison
1989	Laboratory Instructor in Neuropathology for medical students, University of Wisconsin Medical School, Madison
1977 – 1978	Instructor, Pharmacology, University of Colorado Medical School, Denver
1970 – 1973	Tutorial Assistant, Physiological Chemistry for medical students, University of Wisconsin Medical School, Madison

Professional Activities

1998 – 1999	Medical Affairs Committee Chairperson of the Great Lakes Laboratory Network sponsored by Mayo Clinic
1994 – 1999	MD Director of Clinical Chemistry, BMMC/SHE
1995 – 1999	MD Director of Immunology, BMMC/SHE
1994 – 1998	MD Director of Hematopathology, BMMC/SHE
1995 – 1998	MD Director of Flow Cytometry, BMMC/SHE
1994 – 1998	Critical Path Committee, MD Chairperson, BMMC/SHE
1994 – 1997	Research Committee, Co-Director, BMMC
1996 – 1999	Medical Staff Clinical Practice Improvement Committee, BMMC/SHE
1996 – 1999	Point of Care Testing Committee, Chairperson, BMMC
1995 – 1996	Infection Control Committee, BMMC
1997	Ad Hoc Cost Reduction Task Force Committee, BMMC
1994 – 1995	Ad Hoc Quality Assurance Committee, BMMC
1995 – 1999	MD Editor for Laboratory Newsletter, BMMC
1992 – 1993	MD director of Clinical Chemistry, Consultants Lab of WI
1992 – 1993	Medical Staff Quality Assurance Committee, St. Agnes Hospital
1992 – 1993	Continuing Medical Education Committee, St. Agnes Hospital
1991 – 1992	MD Director of Clinical Chemistry, Wenatchee Valley Clinic
1991 – 1992	MD Director of Microbiology, Wenatchee Valley Clinic
1991 – 1992	Infection Control Committee, Wenatchee Valley Clinic
1991 – 1992	Clinical Research Committee, Wenatchee Valley Clinic
1991 – 1992	Computer Utilization Committee, Wenatchee Valley Clinic
1988 – 1990	Blood Product Utilization Review Committee, UW-Madison
1989 – 1990	Resident Editor for University of Wisconsin Hospital Clinical Laboratory Newsletter

Certification and Licensure

National Board of Medical Examiners: 1987
The American Board of Pathology: Diplomat AP/CP, 11/3/93
Medical Licenses: Michigan (4301063871), Wisconsin (28867), Illinois (036086-44, expired), and Washington (27974, expired)

Professional Positions

2001 –present	**Medical Director,** Integrative Healthcare, Blue Heron Academy, Grand Rapids, MI
2000 – 2001	**General Practice**, Integrative Healthcare, Longevity Center of West MI, Rockford, MI
1995 – 2001	**Medical Director**, Sera-Tec Biologicals (plasmapheresis center), Grand Rapids, MI
1999 – 2000	**Medical Director**, Department of Pathology and Laboratory Medicine, West Shore Medical Center, Manistee, MI
1994 – 1999	**Associate Pathologist**, Department of Pathology and Laboratory Medicine, Spectrum Health East (SHE), formerly Blodgett Memorial Medical Center (BMMC), Grand Rapids, MI
1994 – present	**Clinical Assistant Professor**, Department of Pathology, Michigan State University College of Human Medicine, East Lansing, MI
1992 – 1993	**Associate Pathologist**, Department of Pathology, Fond du Lac Pathology Consultants, LTD and Consultants Laboratory of Wisconsin, Inc., Fond du Lac, WI
1991 – 1992	**Associate Pathologist**, Department of Pathology, Wenatchee Valley Clinic, Wenatchee, WA
1978 – 1986	**Assistant/Associate Scientist**, Department of Psychiatry, University of Wisconsin, Madison, WI

Journal Publications

Steele, D.M., **Hegstrand, L.K.,** Julian, T.M., and Storm, F.K.: An Unusual Presentation of Metastatic Squamous Cell Carcinoma of the Vulva. Gynecologic Oncology 39, 218-220, 1990.

Gilbert-Barness, E., **Hegstrand, L.**, Chandra, S., Emery, J.L., Barness, L.A., Franciosi, R., and Huntington, R.: Hazards of Mattresses, Beds, and Bedding in Sudden Death of Infants. Amer J Forensic Ded Path 12, 27-32, 1991.

Partington, C.R., Grave, V.B., and **Hesgtrand, L.K.:** Meningioangiomatosis. Neurorad 12, 549-552, 1991.

Kornguth, S., Gilbert-Barness, E., Langer, E., and **Hegstrand, L.**; Glolgi-Kopsch Silver Study of the Brain of a Patient with Untreated Phenylketonuria, Seizures, and Cortical Blindness. Amer J Med Gen 44, 443-448, 1992.

First or second author on 32 of 39 published articles in referred journals on topics including myelin basic protein, tyrosine hydroxylase, adenylate cyclase, beta-adrenergic receptors, pharmacology of aggressive behavior, and histamine as a neurotransmitter (complete bibliography available upon request).

Abstracts

Abbas, M.M., Warzynski, M.J., and **Hegstrand, L.K.**, Flow Cytometric Detection of Fetal RhD+ Red Blood Cells in RhD- Maternal Cirulation, GRAMEC Research Day, April 1997.

Hegstrand, L.K., Combined Peripheral T-Cell Lymphoma and Hodgkin's Disease Mised Cellularity, Danbury Research Day, May 1994.

Hegstrand, L.K, Miller, R.C., and Koch, D.D.: Fructosamine: Modified Nitroblue Tetrazolium Assay to Improve Clinical Utility. ASCP/CAP, Spring Meeting 1990.

Hegstrand, L.K., Chandra, S., and Gilbert-Barness, E.: Hazards of Mattresses, Beds, and Bedding in Sudden Death of Infants. Society of Pediatric Pathologists Annual Meeting, San Francisco, March 1989.

Hegstrand, L.K., Miller, R.C., and Kock, D.D.: Fructosamine Assay—Confusion and Clarity. Clin. Chem. 34:1271, 1988.

Author on 17 other abstracts on topics described above (complete Bibliography available on request).

Invited Publications
Hegstrand, L.K., A Method Evaluation of the Sanofi Access Progesterone Assay. Lifeline 2: 1, September 1996.

Hegstrand, L.K., Lab Consultant – Fructoseamine. Clin. Chem. News 14: 14-15, 1988.